CONFLUENCE

LANGUAGE ACQUISITION & LANGUAGE DISORDERS

Volume 4

Fred R. Eckman (ed.)

Confluence

CONFLUENCE

LINGUISTICS, L2 ACQUISITION AND SPEECH PATHOLOGY

edited by

FRED R. ECKMAN
University of Wisconsin, Milwaukee

JOHN BENJAMINS PUBLISHING COMPANY
AMSTERDAM/PHILADELPHIA

1993

Library of Congress Cataloging-in-Publication Data

Confluence : linguistics, L2 acquisition, and speech pathology / edited by Fred R. Eckman.

p. cm. -- (Language acquisition & language disorders : ISSN 0925-0123; v. 4)

Papers presented at a conference held Apr. 1989 at the University of Wisconsin-Milwaukee.

Includes bibliographical references.

1. Second language acquisition--Congresses. 2. Language disorders--Congresses. 3. Speech disorders--Congresses. 4. Linguistics--Congresses. I. Eckman, Fred R. II. Series.

P118.2.C65 1993

401'.93--dc20 92-36058

ISBN 90 272 2465 X (Eur.) / 1-55619-237-1 (US) (alk. paper) CIP

John Benjamins Publishing Co. · P.O. Box 75577 · 1070 AN Amsterdam · The Netherlands

John Benjamins North America · 821 Bethlehem Pike · Philadelphia, PA 19118 · USA

Contents

Introduction:

One Approach to the Interaction of Linguistics, Second-language Acquisition, and Speech-language Pathology

Fred R. Eckman

In April of 1989, a symposium on the interaction of linguistics, second language acquisition and speech-language pathology was held on the campus of the University of Wisconsin — Milwaukee. The primary goal of this conference was to provide a forum in which linguists, second-language acquisition specialists and speech-language pathologists could address issues and topics of mutual interest. This volume represents a subset of the papers presented at that symposium.

That these three disciplines impinge on each other in areas of vital importance to each seems to be undeniable. All three fields are concerned with the characterization of language in one form or another; and all deal with the acquisition of language by one segment of the population or another.

Given this context, the primary goal of this collection of papers is to outline some of the areas in which these three disciplines interact. Specifically, it is proposed that an important question, if not the most important question, in the relationship among these three fields is the following:

> What weight or implications do findings in one of the three fields in question have for one or both of the others?

The purpose of raising this question is simply to provide food for thought, since an answer will have to emerge as the relationships among the three disciplines evolve. In view of this, let us, therefore, outline one possible relationship.

Linguistics, as construed by one of the most influential schools of thought in this country, namely, generative grammar, is concerned with the characterization of what a language is, and how it is acquired. Much of the work in this framework centers around the description of the human language faculty, which is assumed to govern language acquisition by children in normal circumstances. Second-language acquisition, on the other hand, deals with the characterization and learning of a language, usually by an adult, when one language is already resident. Speech-language pathology is concerned with the description and treatment of various language disorders in both children and adults, and with the relationship of these so-called disordered languages to normal linguistic systems.

Thus, all of the disciplines deal to some extent with the acquisition of language, and all of the fields overlap with one of the others in the population with which it is concerned. But although these fields of inquiry share a general domain, the specific goals of the individual disciplines are distinct in that each approaches the problem of language description and acquisition from a different perspective. Linguistics and speech-language pathology both concern themselves with primary-language acquisition, but speech-language pathology is concerned with instances in which the acquisition has somehow gone awry or been delayed. Linguistics and second-language acquisition both deal with the description of languages; however, second-language acquisition theory is concerned with learner-languages, or interlanguages. Both speech-language pathology and second-language acquisition deal with language intervention; however, in the case of second-language acquisition, the intervention may be complicated by the fact that there is a language already resident. With each field having developed expertise in its respective area of the problem of language description and acquisition, it seems reasonable that each field has, in principle, something to contribute to, and something to gain from, the others.

The relationship among the three disciplines, in fact, seems to be that of theory to practicum, played out in several directions at once. In general terms, let us define *theory* as being concerned with problems of explanation internal to a given theoretical framework itself, and *practicum* as being involved with solving problems that have more common, every-day implications. The fields of second-language acquisition and speech-language pathology are both comprised of two interrelated branches, one more theoretical, and the other more practical. Second language acquisition encompasses the study of how secondary languages are learned, the theoretical component, and also includes the development of methodologies for teaching these languages, the practicum. Similarly, the field of speech-language pathology, as theory, involves the analysis and explanation of speech and language disorders, and as practicum, the remediation of these disorders through the design and implementation of various intervention techniques and programs. Both of these fields, in the theoretical as well as the pedagogical or clinical areas, make crucial use of principles and constructs from linguistic theories. And under the above definition, it is also fair to say that, relative to linguistics, second-language acquisition and speech-language pathology bear the label of practicum rather than theory.

Ideally, the flow of information among the three disciplines in question would be such that each is informed by work and progress in the others. That such a relationship between theory and practice does not yet exist among the fields being discussed in this volume seems clear. The connection that exists is one in which the theoretical fields inform the practical domains, but the theoretical fields are not informed by the practicums.

Thus, the literature abounds with examples in which both second-language acquisition and speech-language pathology make use of findings and constructs from linguistics. To cite just a few examples, Hyltenstam (1984), Pavesi (1986), and Hawkins (1987) all invoke certain linguistic universals to explain facts about second-language acquisition. Working within a different framework, White (1985) and Flynn (1987) argue for invoking principles of Universal Grammar to account for second-language data. For examples in speech-language pathology, suffice it to note the classic work of McReynolds and Huston (1971), using distinctive features, the recent studies relating phonological knowledge to the rate of learning (Dinnsen 1984), and considerations of some of the potential implications of Government and Binding for speech-language pathology (Leonard and Loeb 1988).

On the other hand, however, there are relatively few and only isolated instances in which it has been proposed that facts from second-language acquisition or speech-language pathology could have a bearing on linguistics. The most explicit case in second-language acquisition is Gass and Ard (1980), in which it is argued that not only do second-language data constitute a viable testing ground for language universals, but in fact these data are a better test than are data from child-language acquisition. As a rule, however, the results of applying linguistic facts and principles to second-language or disordered data do not constitute evidence either for or against those linguistic principles. In short, it is difficult to imagine a linguist, who happens to be a proponent of a certain theory or construct, altering or abandoning that construct on the basis of evidence obtained in the clinic or the classroom. In fact, in view of apparent counterevidence to linguistic generalizations from, say, second-language data, it is not suggested that the generalizations should be revised or abandoned even by those who did not propose the generalizations.

As an illustration of this point, let us consider an example from the second-language acquisition literature. The principle involved is the Accessible Hierarchy (Keenan and Comrie 1977), which attempts to characterize the types of relative clause constructions found in the world's languages. This hierarchy, shown below, predicts that if a language can form a relative clause by relativizing an NP from a given position, x, on the hierarchy, that language can necessarily form relative clauses by relativizing NP's in all positions higher than x, but that such a language cannot necessarily relativize NP from positions lower than x. Thus, for example, a language which can form relative clauses by relativizing the indirect object NP, can necessarily relativize the direct object and subject NP's, but such a language may not be able to relativize an NP which is the object of a preposition, genitive or object of a comparative.

(1) Accessibility Hierarchy
Subj
Dir obj
Ind Obj
Obj of Prep
Gen
Obj of a Comparative

This hierarchy, or parts of it, have been invoked to explain data from second-language acquisition in a number of different studies (Gass 1979; Hyltenstam 1984; Pavesi 1986). What is of interest is that the second-language data do not conform completely to the hierarchy, or stated differently, the hierarchy is not completely supported by the data. For Gass' findings, the Genitive position was ranked higher than the Direct object position; for Hyltenstam the Object of the preposition ranked higher than the Indirect object; and for both Hyltenstam and Pavesi, the Genitive position ranked last, lower than the object of a comparative particle. Despite these findings, no one questioned the Accessibility Hierarchy, or suggested that the ranking of the positions should be changed.

This relationship between theory and practice does not hold in all disciplines. A situation in which findings in two separate fields impinge on the other, where one can be said to be theoretical and the other can be said to be practical, is outlined in a paper by Ritchie (1978). He considers the relationship between biological science and clinical medicine, and argues that theories of pathology developed by biological science have a direct bearing on how diseases are treated clinically. Likewise, the results obtained by such clinical treatment serve as a test for the theory of the disease. Ritchie goes on to argue that this relationship between the theory and the practicum is at least in part responsible for the great advancement that has been made by medical science in the treatment of infectious diseases.

Given that the situation among the three disciplines under discussion in this volume is one in which theory unidirectionally informs practicum, the question arises as to whether this relationship is a necessary one. Referring back to Ritchie's example, it is not in the nature of things that all relationships between theory and practicum must be this way. Therefore, the issue becomes, is it in the nature of the theories and practicums in question that the information flow must be unidirectional?

It does not appear that one could make the case that data from secondary languages and speech-language pathology could not inform linguistics, because such data would constitute special cases as a result of the controlled or experimental situations in which the data were obtained. When one considers the situation in established sciences, such as chemistry or physics, one sees that chemists and physicists are generally less concerned with phenomena that occur naturally, and much more concerned with facts observed under the special or controlled conditions of the laboratory.

While it is admittedly premature to expect some fundamental insight or answer to this question, the goal of this volume is to open discussion on the issue. The papers are grouped into three general areas, namely, those dealing with: (1) linguistics and second language acquisition, (2) linguistics and speech-language pathology, and (3) second-language acquisition and speech-language pathology.

Turning first to linguistics and second-language acquisition, the issue of the implications of evidence in one field for arguments and claims in the other is addressed in the papers by Flynn and Rutherford. Both of these authors argue for a "two-way street" of communication between linguistics and second-language acquisition theory; one in which second-language specialists inform as well as are informed by linguistics. Rutherford makes the point that the goals of both disciplines are woven together in the issue of learnability. Flynn carries the matter a little farther: she argues that facts about second language acquisition fall into the proper domain of linguistic theory. According to Flynn, grammars learned by second-language learners are governed by the principles of Universal Grammar (UG).

This notion that UG governs the grammars of secondary languages is echoed by other contributions in this first section. Klein considers what she terms the null preposition phenomenon, and proposes that this is a stage in the acquisition of preposition stranding. Platt addresses the question of the Null Subject Parameter of UG in a study of Vietnamese and Spanish learners of English. Her results present some problems for previous analyses. And Martohardjono and Gair take up the issue of the availability of UG in second language acquisition. They argue that showing the absence of some principle of UG in second language acquisition does not mean that UG is unavailable to the learner. Rather, they argue that the conditions necessary for the application of certain UG principles may not be met.

The other two papers in the first section deal with the notion of markedness in second-language acquisition. Balhorn looks at various notions of markedness to determine whether non-native speakers of English produce marked structures with the same frequency as native speakers. And Archibald considers the notion of markedness in the acquisition of stress placement from the point view of learnability. More specifically he raises several questions, including (1) whether the native language parameter is transferred, (2) how much data are required to trigger resetting the parameter in question, and (3) whether such triggering is the result of a mismatch between a learner's perception and production. In the second group of papers, which deals with the relationship between linguistics and speech-language pathology, the contributions by Dinnsen and Connell address disordered speech in children, and the one by Chen treats language disorders in adults.

Dinnsen proposes that the domain of misarticulated speech constitutes part of the domain of linguistics, because, he argues, the data from misarticulating children can be accounted for by existing linguistic principles. This suggests, in turn, that misarticulated data can be explained through the extension of linguistic theory to misarticulated speech, where extending the theory in this way results in no loss of generality. He goes on to claim that, although misarticulated speech may be "deviant" when considered in relation to the ambient language, it is not deviant when looked at with respect to the range of possible variation among languages. The paper by Connell echoes the same theme. He argues that only language intervention which is grounded in a theory of language acquisition stands to yield fruitful results. Thus, for him, linguistic theory has definite implications for language remediation. He builds his case using data from specific language impaired (SLI) children, citing differences in how these children seem to acquire language relative to normal children.

The paper in this section that deals with adult speakers is by Chen. In a very interesting contribution, she considers the problem of morphology in aphasics from the viewpoint of two different models: the syndrome-dominant model and the languge-dominant model. She tests the predictions of these models, comparing facts from Chinese aphasics to those from English-speaking aphasics, and she concludes that morphological differences between languages affect aphasic symptoms.

In the final section, which deals with the relationship between speech-language pathology and second language acquisition, Damico discusses the similar histories of the two disciplines, tracing them through their early concern with "successful" language performance, to their structuralist orientation in the middle part of this century, on to the integrative, socio-linguistic approach of the last two decades. Damico points out that there have also been significant differences in the development the two fields, and that each discipline is in a position to benefit from the other.

Gierut, in her contribution, makes the same point quite convincingly, citing evidence from experimental studies. After discussing some of the ways in which speech-language pathology has benefitted from developments in second-language acquisition, Gierut addresses the ways in which second language acquisition could benefit from the methodology used in some studies in speech-language pathology. Specifically, she proposes the use of single-subject designs, a research design which has been used extensively by speech-language pathologists. In a single-subject design, treatment is performed on individuals rather than on groups in such a way that the individuals serve as their own controls. Gierut goes on to discuss some of the advantages of this methodology.

The paper by Hardy is a study employing these single-subject methods on an adult, second-language learner. She attempted to answer a number of questions about the subject's interlanguage phonological system, such as which phonemes are learned first, what generalization takes place, and whether the subject retains what is learned from the training. One interesting aspect of this paper is that Hardy found several differences between her L2 subject and the findings of similar studies performed on misarticulating children.

The final paper in this section, the contribution by Kempler and van Lancker, deals with the performance of stroke patients and ESL learners on both idioms (what is termed "familiar language") and novel phrases. The authors found a number of differences between the stroke patients and the L2 learners, suggesting familiar and non-familiar language are both different and learned independently of each other.

In sum, the point has been argued that all of the disciplines in question impinge on each other in important ways. It would be difficult to imagine how someone could seriously defend the position that the three disciplines are not interrelated. Despite this, there has been relatively little, formal interaction. It is hoped that this volume will open a discussion that will be both fruitful and on-going.

References

Connell, P. 1986. "Acquisition of Semantic Relations by Language-disordered Children: Comprehension or Production". *Journal of Speech and Hearing Research* 29.384-397.

Dinnsen, D. 1984. "Methods and Empirical Issues in Analyzing Functional Misarticulations. Elbert, Dinnsen and Weismer 1984.

Elbert, M., D. Dinnsen and G. Weismer, eds. 1984. *Phonological Theory and the Misarticulating Child*. Rockville, MD: American Speech-Language-Hearing Association.

Flynn, S. 1987. *A Parametric Approach to L2 Acquisition*. Dordrecht: D. Reidel Publishing Co.

Gass, S. 1979. "Language Transfer and Universal Grammatical Relations". *Language Learning* 29.327-344.

Gass, S and J. Ard. 1980. "L2 Data: Their Relevance for Language Universals". *TESOL Quarterly* 14.443-452.

Gierut, J. 1986. "Sound change: A Phonemic Split in a Misarticulating Child". *Applied Psycholoinguistics* 7.57-68.

Hawkins, J. 1987. "Implicational Universals as Predictors of Language Acquisition". *Linguistics* 25.453-473.

Hyltenstam, K. 1984. "The Use of Typological Markedness Conditions as Predictors in Second Language Acquisition: The Case of Pronominal Copies in Relative Clauses". *Second Languages* ed. by R. Andersen, 39-58. Rowley, MA: Newbury House Publishers.

Keenan, E. and B. Comrie. 1977. "Noun Phrase Accessibility and Universal Grammar". *Linguistic Inquiry* 8.63-99.

Leonard, L. and D.F. Loeb. 1988. "Government-Binding Theory and Some of its Applications: A Tutorial." *Journal of Speech and Hearing Research* 31.515-524.

McReynolds, L. and K. Huston. 1971. "A Distinctive Feature Analysis of Children's Misarticulations". *Journal of Speech and Hearing Disorders* 36.155-166.

Pavesi, M. 1986. "Markedness, Discoursal Modes and Relative Clause Formation in a Formal and an Informal Context". *Studies in Second Language Acquisition* 8.38-55.

Ritchie, W. 1978. "Introduction: Theory and Practice in Second Language Research and Teaching". *Second Language Acquisition Research: Issues and Implications* ed. by W. Ritchie, 1-9. New York: Academic Press.

White, L. 1985. "The 'Pro-drop' Parameter in Adult Second Language Acquisition". *Language Learning* 35.47-62.

Linguistics and SLA

Linguistics and SLA:

The Two-Way Street Phenomenon

William E. Rutherford
University of Southern California

There are a number of perspectives from which one can view the relationship of the field of linguistics to the relatively new field of second language acquisition (SLA).[1] One can, for example, simply recite the chronology of all linguistic references that have figured in SLA research over its twenty-five year history. Or one might choose to focus specifically on those approaches to the study of grammar that have informed SLA research during these two decades — approaches such as those of Greenbergian typology, Chomskyan UG, language function à la Givón, Thompson, etc., earlier versions of transformational grammar, language variation à la Bickerton, Bailey, Labov, etc. Or one might wish to single out the most significant pieces of SLA research that have emerged during this time and review the extent to which a command of linguistics is a contributor to that significance. Any of these perspectives, and no doubt others as well, could easily constitute the framework for developing a paper that would adequately address the question of the relationship of SLA to linguistics. Notice, however, that these ways of approaching the task all imply that the nature of the relationship to be discussed is not necessarily one obtaining between co-equal disciplines. Rather, the implication is that this relationship is one between an informing discipline — namely linguistics — and an informed discipline — namely SLA. In fact it is quite common to find SLA identified as a kind of "applied linguistics" itself.[2]

As is probably obvious by now, I want to challenge this very common unidirectional presumption vis-à-vis linguistics and second language acquisition. It is a misperception long in need of correction, and some of that correction is already implicit in ongoing work. Therefore, in terms both of the kinds of SLA research currently being conducted and of what kinds we can expect to see in the years ahead, the only fair way to characterize the linguistics/SLA relationship is as a two-way street. That is, both disciplines are, at least potentially, mutually informing and mutually informed. I would like first to consider how the notion of a two-way street phenomenon has come about (for it didn't start out that way), then to take stock of its current manifestations, and finally to hazard a few guesses as to other areas where light may well be shed through the energy of this SLA/linguistics symbiosis. In fact, I will suggest at the end that even the "two-way street" metaphor is not quite apt either.

In a very real sense, the evolution of a bi-directional SLA/linguistics relationship is co-extensive with the development of SLA as a theory-grounded discipline. And the kinds of theoretical questions posed by SLA researchers over the field's history describe, also in a very real sense, the kinds of linguistics that have played a role in that development. In looking back, how long have we seen an SLA discipline in which it is possible to raise true theoretical issues? For a lot of us perhaps, the onset of this development coincides with the fundamental shift of perspective in the late sixties from language learning as a behavioristic phenomenon to language learning as a mentalistic one. Central to this shift was the notion that elements of the language learner's own cognition play a crucial role in his attainment of target language criteria. Investigation of those elements thus quickly became the principal aim of SLA research at that time, and this for many meant discerning a general order in the emergence in learner production of a small class of bound morphemes and grammatical functors. Although some benefits from this procedure did accrue to the field, from a linguistic standpoint (and with the advantage of hindsight) nothing explanatory was being claimed at all, simply because ordering the adhoc assemblage of unrelated items in question fell out from no theory of anything.I think now that what we saw then was the curious result of attempts to grapple with an (unfamiliar) psycholinguistic problem using the tools of outmoded linguistic structuralism. The field at that point had, in a sense, its linguistic foot in the past and its psycholinguistic foot in the present.

Another way of characterizing the status of the field of SLA at that point in time is to adopt a pair of metaphors cited a decade ago by Huebner (1983). Acquisition research was in transition — moving away from perception of adult language learning as "running an open field race" and toward perception of it as "negotiating a maze." As an (unconstrained) open field race, SLA was in a position to be neither informed nor informing with respect to linguistics. With SLA as the (constrained) negotiation of a maze, the stage is finally set for development of some kind of SLA/linguistics partnership.

Setting the stage is one thing; letting something happen upon that stage is quite another, however. What we saw played out on stage at the beginning was a drama in which linguistics was essentially the informing discipline, SLA the informed, along with a general unstated assumption that this unidirectionality was a quite natural state of affairs. I'm referring here to the linguistic events surrounding one of the earliest of the serious research questions posed in SLA — viz. the interlanguage hypothesis (Selinker 1972) — and its subsequent revitalization (Adjémian 1976).[3] The interlanguage hypothesis held that interim learner language qualifies as natural language in that it is internally systematic at any given point in its development. Adjémian's contribution was to redefine that systematicity in terms of a characteristic that set interlanguage apart from the rest of natural language — namely, its susceptibility to "permeation" by elements from both source and target language. What makes Adjémian's work of the mid-seventies stand out for us is that he was one of the very few L2 researchers of the time who both had a good grasp of grammatical theory and was able to bring it into his work on SLA. His contribution was to refine the IL hypothesis to a point where claims of IL internal systematicity were actually testable — e.g. consistent transfer of verb subcategorization features, as in subject-to-object raising for target French.

The IL hypothesis was the first of a series of important hypotheses concerning SLA that collectively and conveniently serve as framework for viewing the linguistics/L2 relationship. If IL was claimed to satisfy the necessary criteria for identification as natural language, it had not yet — unlike the rest of the world's languages — been recognized by formal grammarians as a repository of data to be culled in support of particular theoretical stances. That was not to happen for yet another decade.

What we saw instead was in a sense the reverse: a succession of studies by L2 researchers designed, in essence, to test out the IL hypothesis through recourse to various principles of formal linguistics. Ritchie's (1978) study concluded tentatively, for example, that IL obeys the "right-roof constraint" of universal grammar (more recently argued as being subsumed by the principle of subjacency).[4] Schmidt's (1980) study concluded that IL obeys universal constraints on the surface orders of coordinate structures.

Eckman's (1981) phonological study concluded that although the IL "schwa paragoge" phenomenon arises solely in a language contact situation, it does not violate any known phonological principles.[5]

If IL meets the qualifications for membership in the great class of natural languages, it was only reasonable that one should have then been curious about the status of its acquisition vis-à-vis that of the mother tongue. That is, factoring out the obvious circumstantial differences, are language acquisition in childhood and in adulthood cognitively indistinguishable? This curiosity led to the next serious research question being considered here: the L2=L1 hypothesis. Let it be noted, however, that even at this point in SLA's historical development the L2=L1 hypothesis is one formulated by the L2 researchers, not their L1 counterparts. In fact, the question of L2/L1 relationship was still apparently not even of interest to L1 theoreticians and grammarians. This observation is most strikingly underscored through inspection of perhaps the most widely cited collection of seminal papers on the language acquisition topic — namely, the volume edited by Wanner and Gleitman (1982) titled Language Acquisition: the State of the Art. Not only are there no papers on adult language acquisition among the fourteen assembled in that volume, but also there is not even any reference made to language acquisition in adulthood, nor for that matter to child second language acquisition either. The index to Wanner and Gleitman (1982) contains no such entries and among the thirty-four pages of cumulative references there is not a single citation to be found for SLA — and this was 1982. One has to conclude that, from the perspective of researchers outside of SLA, L2 was but a mere circumstantial variant of L1. Hence, the term "language acquisition" in Wanner and Gleitman needed no ordinal-number qualification.

I think it is not unfair to say that from the standpoint of L2 research L2=L1 is a hypothesis, while for most L1 researchers L2=L1 is a foregone conclusion. There are two ways that I know of to reveal that such a conclusion has been reached. One of them is through silence, as in the absence of any reference to L2 in the Wanner and Gleitman volume just mentioned. The other is to take an acquisition model derived exclusively upon L1 data and simply extend its coverage to L2 without acknowledging, let alone addressing, the crucial questions that are now at the forefront of current SLA research. We have a good example of this too. A recent special issue of Applied Psycholinguistics (Snow and Locke 1987) is entirely devoted to explorations of bilingualism within MacWhinney's "Competition Model," which is claimed by its proponents to be able to embrace acquisition of both L1 and L2, which supposedly differ only by virtue of the fact that L2 is susceptible to L1 transfer. Simply factoring out transfer thus erases any L1/L2 distinctions since, as MacWhinney (1987:317) states: "for those areas of L2 where transfer has not occurred, the L2 learner is in the position of the L1 learner and must simply learn from scratch". Similarly, another of the papers in this same volume states naively at one point that "with enough second language exposure, [L2 learner] performance can become indistinguishable from that of native speakers" (McDonald 1987:412).[6]

The facts concerning acquisition of one's native language and the final state attained by the adult grammar has delimited the research area of interest to formal grammarians as well. As with Wanner and Gleitman, the volume edited by Tavakolian (1981) titled Language Acquisition and Linguistic Theory likewise takes the word "acquisition" to mean "by children learning their mother tongue," and the editor's preface alludes to the two-way street phenomenon with respect to formal linguistics and L1: "This volume focuses on the significance of language-acquisition studies to the construction of theories of adult language" (Tavakolian 1981:vii). As long as the primary interest of linguistics was in the final-state grammars of adult *native* speakers and how such grammars are attained, there was of course no need to worry about how the picture might be complicated by a vast population of adult non-native learners whose "final state" grammars not only invariably stopped short of target criteria but also neither displayed cross-learner homogeneity nor were even attained in accord with the learning principles adduced for native-language acquisition. This state of affairs was not to last forever, but change was slow in coming.

Until the early eighties, the idea that IL data might be of value to empirical research in formal linguistics had not apparently occurred to anyone not already devoted to the study of SLA. One of the first demonstrated changes in this perception that I know of happened at the conference on language universals and second language acquisition held at USC early in 1982, whose proceedings appeared in print two years later (Rutherford 1984). The intent of the conference organizers was that L2 researchers and grammatical theorists should address, each from his/her own perspective, the subject of language universals and their relation to adult language acquisition, with commentary provided from the other discipline. The novel aspect in all this was of course that non-SLA oriented researchers should be drawing upon SLA sources to support positions with respect to grammatical theory. Thus, Givon (1984) used L2 data from a 1979 transcript of Schumann's to argue for certain universals of topic marking. Bickerton (1984) used L2 findings from Huebner (1983) to argue for his "bioprogram hypothesis." And Comrie (1984) used L2 findings from Gass (1979) to argue for the value of L2 data in establishing cross-linguistic implicational relationships such as those manifested in accessibility hierarchies. A passage from the Comrie study best captures the essence of the conference organizers' intent: "...the literature has pointed to a number of ways in which research on language universals and research on second language acquisition can benefit one another" (Comrie 1984:11). The "universals" referred to in the Comrie quote were those to be ascertained by virtue of sampling among large quantities of the world's languages — i.e. universals derived within the Greenbergian research paradigm. And of course the state of SLA research in 1982 was such that this was the only kind of language universal figuring in L2 studies up to that time; hence the conference was not a forum for focus on universals relevant to the Chomskyan research paradigm.

Focus of that kind within an open forum was to come three and a half years later, at the 1985 MIT conference on linguistic theory and second language acquisition organized by Suzanne Flynn and Wayne O'Neil. Although the conference rubric mentioned only "linguistic theory," it was clear, both from the conference venue and from the roster of invited participants, that "linguistic theory" meant Universal Grammar (UG, or more specifically, parameterized UG). Moreover, the conference was not intended as a forum to debate the status of UG vis-à-vis SLA. That status was to be taken for granted. Rather, the purpose of the conference, in the words of its organizers, "at its most general level, was to examine the extent to which a theory of UG could be useful in explaining the L2 acquisition process" (Flynn and O'Neil 1988:1). Indeed, only one paper presented, Clahsen's study of verb placement acquisition by children and adults, explicitly denied a central influence of UG upon emerging adult L2 grammars. The rest accepted, to varying degrees, a definite role for UG.

A mere assumption that UG is operant in SLA does not by itself of course tell us anything about a possible bi-directionality of linguistics/SLA interest. Although Flynn and O'Neil, in their own words, also "sought to examine the extent to which L2 acquisition findings might uniquely contribute to the development of a theory of UG" (Flynn and O'Neil 1988:2), the conference and its published proceedings, valuable though they are, largely served to elucidate facets of adult language learning through the *mediation* of UG and the empirical consequences for L2 that arise from working within such a theoretical framework.[7]

The use of SLA to support different approaches to questions of grammatical theory were of course not limited to the proceedings of the two conferences just discussed. Another example concerns the attention devoted to implicational universals, beginning with Eckman's paper from the SLA side at the 1982 USC conference, but continuing with Hawkins (1987) from the linguistics side, and most recently Eckman, Moravcsik and Wirth (1989) from both sides. Eckman (1984) demonstrated the value of implicational universals in predicting where apparent violations may occur in a language contact situation. Hawkins (1987) uses L2 (and L1) data, some of it drawn from Eckman's study, to argue for the theoretical status of implicational universals. Thus, implicationals, at this point in the scenario that I'm sketching, had figured in two different purposes: SLA used them to validate the IL hypothesis; linguistics used SLA to validate implicationals. With Eckman, Moravcsik and Wirth (1989) the two purposes, so to speak, coalesce. In that paper, titled "Interlanguages: how language-like are they?", the authors arrive at a principle identified by them as the Structural Conformity Hypothesis, which they argue can extend the relevance of implicational facts to two kinds of non-primary language — child L1 and adult L2 — and to phylogenetic as well as to ontogenetic development. Implicationals are thus imbued here with their heaviest explanatory force and SLA has been the major impetus in the authors' extension of that force to the language phenomena just mentioned.

If the 1982 USC conference saw SLA as a contributor to theories of typological universals and the 1985 MIT conference saw SLA as a contributor to the theory of a parameterized Universal Grammar, it was to be only two years later than that — the 1987 Stanford conference organized by Thom Huebner and Charles Ferguson — when SLA would draw the attention of linguists working within still other theoretical models. Thus, a Relational Grammar perspective was represented by Carol Rosen, natural morphology by Joan Bybee, "functional linguistics" by Cooreman and Kilborn, variation theory by John Rickford, prosodic phonology by Irene Vogel, and so on. The very title of the Stanford conference is important, for it captures quite well the transition state which SLA had by then attained — Second Language Acquisition: Contributions and Challenges to Linguistic Theory, and I underscore the word "challenges."

One might notice now, if one hasn't already, that the events surrounding these various conferences, etc. on the general theme of SLA and linguistics, and the kinds of research question posed, start to present a pattern. The earliest phase of second language acquisition as an emerging discipline was one in which SLA, in its efforts to explore the implications of the IL hypothesis, drew substantially from descriptive work in linguistics. Next we find grammarians supporting one or another theoretical position in linguistics by drawing for the first time from SLA research. Then we have the first suggestion from SLA that maybe the characteristics of adult language acquisition are such that they could not only offer grist for the linguistics mill but throw in an occasional monkey wrench as well. And through most of it all, there is the absence of any notable research in which cognitive aspects of language acquisition in childhood and in adulthood are linked in any serious way — absent in child L1 research because L1 and L2 are supposedly the same; absent in adult L2 research because L1 and L2 are supposedly different. We thus have three major research strands — child L1, adult L2, and formal linguistics — somewhat frayed strands that often get tangled but that are about to be woven into a braid.[8] The braid is "learnability."

Until very recently, most L1 and L2 acquisition research concerned with grammatical competence has taken the form of descriptive studies documenting the emergence of target syntactic features. One of the results of these kinds of studies was the purported similarity of L2 to L1 with respect to the orders which these features were seen to manifest and to the developmental stages adducible from the orders. But this of course tells us nothing about how the grammars incorporating such features get learned — or don't get learned. Since we do not know what factors (perhaps even accidental ones) have given rise to the fragments of parallel grammatical development that have been tabulated, it is research findings in the learnability sector that constitute the litmus test for fundamental research questions of primary and non-primary language convergence or divergence.

The learnability issue then is at least one crucial point of intersection for the study of final-state formal grammars, the study of how and why children unfailingly attain them, and the study of how and why these same children, having reached adulthood, unfailingly do not attain them. Notice the important interdependencies here. One of them was stated almost ten years ago by Wexler and Culicover (1980:596): "One can't have a theory of how something is acquired without a theory of what that something is". There is another interdependency that can be articulated here and now: We can't have an adequate theory of how something is acquired while at the same time ignoring the fact that such acquisition does not go on forever. Accounting for those different final-state grammars, in childhood and in adulthood, is therefore one place where it all comes together, so to speak.

It's worth pointing out that we've already had the first of what will doubtless be a succession of conference events (including, of course, the symposium represented by the papers in this volume) for at least trying to bring it all together — namely, the special section on Universal Grammar at the 1989 Second Language Research Forum (SLRF) in Los Angeles (Eubank 1991). Here we had grammatical theorists, L2 acquisition researchers, and L1 acquisition researchers (with some filling more than one role) all addressing questions of whether or not adult learners fall back upon an initial-state UG or UG only via its L1 instantiation, whether or not they have access to anything other than principles of general cognition, or even whether or not the ineluctable fact of adult failure forces one to re-examine the very concept of UG itself. And although for the most part it is acquisition of syntax that has headed the research agendas (and has therefore been the focus of this paper), a shift of attention to the lexicon may well be in the offing. As Aitchison (1988:357) put it, "...L2 acquisition, where a lexicon has to be built from scratch, is likely to provide valuable hypotheses about principles which may underlie the mental lexicon, and the interaction of the lexicon with the syntax".[9] As these issues continue to be confronted in the near future, I should imagine that the existing sharp lines of demarcation between the disciplines in question will become more blurred, such that it will eventually be appropriate to start thinking more in terms of a discipline called simply "language acquisition," with no ordinal number appendage. When that happens, the apt descriptive metaphor will be not "two-way street" but rather "major intersection." It might take awhile for us to get there.

Notes

1. Other recent papers addressing this topic are Lightbown and White (1987), Gregg (1986), Sharwood Smith (1988), and Rutherford (1988).

2. Much as, several decades ago, formal instruction (for teaching a language) was identified as applied linguistics. Given that the development of the field of SLA grew out of language teaching concerns, the contemporary view of SLA as applied linguistics should therefore not be too surprising. Newmeyer and Weinberger (1988:41) make no bones about it: "[SLA] is an applied science".

   We think this way at USC as well, in that within our own linguistics department we have been offering students either a "general" program or an "applied" program, the latter being the repository of SLA research, whose faculty are called "applied." I myself am so categorized by most of my departmental colleagues and when my recent promotion came through I was given the title "Professor of Applied Linguistics."

3. See Selinker and Lamendella (1981) for an updating of the IL hypothesis.

4. See Schachter (1989) for extensive criticism of the Ritchie study.

5. In Bley-Vroman (1983) we were given a sharp reminder that in other SLA studies the IL hypothesis was susceptible to underming by the "comparative fallacy" — viz. a lapse into learner language analysis and quantification carried out with reference to target language norms rather than to IL production considered *sui generis*. In all practicality, however, it may be well nigh impossible in conducting IL research to avoid comparative-fallacy contamination, at least in some small measure.

6. It is worth noting that of the five papers assembled in Snow and Locke (1987), two of the three that are written by non-SLA researchers contain virtually no reference at all to the rich SLA research literature, current or otherwise, and the handful of SLA references contained in the third paper are more than a decade old.

7. An exception would be Liceras (1988:199), who wrote of "the possibility of using evidence from L2 acquisition for determining the nature of the boundary between the core and peripheral systems in grammars".

8. I ignore here some obvious other strands such as language processing.

9. The great importance of the lexicon has been stressed by others as well. Wexler and Manzini (1987:47), for example, point out that parameterization is ultimately lexical: "...it has long been recognized by linguistic theory that the lexicon states much or most of the idiosyncracies in a language". Likewise Wasow (1985:203) from an acquisition perspective: "The problem of acquiring a language...reduces largely to learning the meanings of words. There is more to it, of course, such as discovering the basic order of constituents, determining what the bounding nodes are, and learning which verbs trigger S'-deletion (such as *seem* and *believe* in English), and so on. In the canonical cases, however, sentence structure is a projection of the semantics of words".

References

Adjemian, C. 1976. "On the Nature of Interlanguage Systems". *Language Learning* 26.297-320.

Aitchison, J. 1988. "All Paths Lead to the Mental Lexicon. Flynn and O'Neil 1988.346-361.

Bickerton, D. 1984. "The Language Bioprogram Hypothesis and Second Language Acquisition". Rutherford 1984.141-161.

Bley-Vroman, R. 1983. "The Comparative Fallacy in Interlanguage Studies: The Case of Systematicity". *Language Learning* 33.1-17

Comrie, B. 1984. "Why Linguists Need Language Acquirers". Rutherford 1984.11-29.

Eckman, F. 1981. "On the Naturalness of Interlanguage Phonological Rules". *Language Learning* 31.195-216.

Eckman, F. 1984. "Universals, Typologies and Interlanguage". Rutherford 1984.79-105.

Eckman, F., E. Moravcsik, and J. Wirth. 1989. "Interlanguages: How Language-like Are They?" *Milwaukee Studies in Language* 2.59-83.

Eubank, L., ed. 1991. *Point Counterpoint: Universal Grammar in the Second Language*. Amsterdam: John Benjamins.

Flynn, S., and W. O'Neil, eds. 1988. *Linguistic Theory in Second Language Acquisition*. Dordrecht: Kluwer Academic Publishers.

Gass, S. 1979. "Language Transfer and Universal Grammatical Relations". *Language Learning* 29.327-344.

Givón, T. 1984. Universals of Discourse and Second Language Acquisition. Rutherford 1984.109-136.

Gregg, K. 1986. "Linguistic Perspectives on Second Language Acquisition: What Could They Be, and Where Can We Get Some?" Unpublished manuscript, Matsuyama University.

Hawkins, J. 1987. "Implicational Universals as Predictors of Language Acquisition. *Linguistics* 25.453-473.

Huebner, T. 1983. *A Longitudinal Analysis of the Acquisition of English*. Ann Arbor: Karoma.

Liceras, J. 1988. "L2 Learnability: Delimiting the Domain of Core Grammar as Distinct from the Marked Periphery". Flynn and O'Neil 1988.199-224

Lightbown, P. and L. White. 1987. "The Influence of Linguistic Theories on Language Acquisition Research: Description and Explanation". *Language Learning* 37.483-510.

MacWhinney, B. 1987. "Applying the Competition Model to Bilingualism". Snow and Locke 1987.

McDonald, J. 1987. "Sentence Interpretation in Bilingual Speakers of English and Dutch. Snow and Locke 1987.

Newmeyer, F. and S. Weinberger. 1988. "The Ontogenesis of the Field of Second Language Learning Research". Flynn and O'Neil 1988.34-45.

Ritchie, W. 1978. "The Right-roof Constraint in Adult-acquired Language. *Second Language Acquisition Research: Issues and Implications*. ed. by W. Ritchie, 33-63. New York: Academic Press.

Rutherford, W., ed. 1984. *Language Universals and Second Language Acquisition*. Amsterdam: John Benjamins.

Rutherford, W. 1988. "Grammatical Theory and L2 Acquisition: A Brief Overview". Flynn and O'Neil 1984.404-416.

Schachter, J. 1989. "A New Look at an Old Classic". *Second Language Research* 5.30-42.

Schmidt, M. 1980. "Coordinate Structures and Language Universals in Interlanguage". *Language Learning* 30.397-416.

Selinker, L. 1972. "Interlanguage". *International Review of Applied Linguistics* 10.209-231.

Selinker, L. and J. Lamendella. 1981. "Updating the Interlanguage Hypothesis". *Studies in Second Language Acquisition* 3.201-220.

Sharwood Smith, M. 1988. "On the Role of Linguistic Theory in Explanations of Second Language Developmental Grammars". Flynn and O'Neil 1988.173-198.

Snow, C., and J. Locke eds. 1987. *The Competition Model and Bilingualism*. Special issue of *Applied Psycholinguistics*. Vol.8, no.4.

Tavakolian, S., ed. 1981. *Language Acquisition and Linguistic Theory*. Cambridge, MA: MIT Press.

Wanner, E. and L. Gleitman, eds. 1982. *Language Acquisition: The State of the Art*. Cambridge: Cambridge University Press.

Wasow, T. 1985. "Postscript". *Lectures on Contemporary Syntactic Theories* by P. Sells, 192-205 Stanford, CA: Center for the Study of Language and Information.

Wexler, K. and P. Culicover. 1980. *Formal Principles of Language Acquisition*. Cambridge, MA: MIT Press.

Wexler, K., and R. Manzini. 1987. "Parameters and Learnability Theory". *Parameter Setting* ed. by T. Roeper and E. Williams, 41-76. Dordrecht: D. Reidel Publishing Company.

Interactions between L2 Acquisition and Linguistic Theory

Suzanne Flynn
Massachusetts Institute of Technology

Introduction

This paper focuses both on the implications of linguistic theory for second language (L2) learning and the implications of L2 learning for linguistic theory. Development of a full understanding of the L2 learning process and of an explanatory theory of linguistics are intimately related. If linguistic theory is to characterize how language learning is possible in the human organism, then it must make reference to L2 learning. Traditionally, this language learning process has often been ignored by theoretical linguistics (although see recent discussion in Chomsky 1988a,b); this has resulted in the development of a theory of language and language learning which, in spite of its claims, is non-explanatory for the language learning process in general.[2]

At the same time, if a full understanding of second language learning is to be attained, then this must take place within a framework that makes reference to the abstract generalizations provided by theoretical linguistics. Failure to do so could result in the development of theories of L2 acquisition that themselves will prove non-explanatory and which will keep the field forever outside central domains of theoretical linguistics and related areas of cognitive science. It will also lead to the development of non-unified theories of language acquisition in general.

Within recent years significant advances have been made in theoretical linguistics, especially with regard to the theory of principles and parameters within a theory of Universal Grammar (UG); important advances have also been made in the study of the L2 learning process. We are, thus, now in a position to investigate and attempt to understand the relationship between these two domains in a more meaningful manner. More precisely, we can now examine to what extent theoretical linguistics can inform the study of adult L2 acquisition and how evidence gleaned from this study can constrain theories of language and the mind.

Focus of this paper

In this paper, I argue that there exists a very direct and important relationship between linguistic theory, specifically a theory of UG, and adult L2 learning. Specifically, in spite of the differences that we know to exist between the adult L2 learner and the child L1 learner, namely advanced cognitive development, and knowledge of at least one language, the adult solves certain aspects of the language acquisition problem in a manner comparable to that for the child L1 learner. Specifically, the adult L2 acquisition process is constrained by a set of language principles isolated in L1 acquisition. This means that the adult is sensitive to many of the same dimensions of language organization that the child L1 learner is and that establishing these dimensions is necessary in terms of working out other aspects of the new target grammar. These dimensions of language grammar are given to us by a theory of UG and they are not limited by L1 instantiations of UG alone. [3]

Thus, in this paper I will argue, consistent with a theory of UG that the basic biologically driven foundations for language learning observed in child L1 acquisition also hold in adult L2 learning. This means that UG as a theory of language significantly constrains L2 learning. I will also argue that the study of L2 learning can significantly constrain the formation of formal theories of language.[4]

Background

Universal Grammar

The most explicit theory of the human competence for language and its acquisition has been proposed by Chomsky. As suggested in (1), this theory of UG attempts to discover and define the fundamental principles and parameters of all possible natural languages. Principles determine properties of language common to all languages; parameters specify a finite number of principled ways languages differ from each other.

As a theory of the human mind, UG determines what is biologically programmed for language in the child at birth. As such, it represents a formalization of the "language faculty" as an identifiable system of the mind/brain (Chomsky 1988c).

(1) Universal Grammar and the Initial State:

> The initial state of the language faculty consists of a collection of subsystems, or modules as they are called, each of which is based on certain very general principles. Each of these principles admits of a certain very limited possibility of variation. We may think of the system as a complex network, associated with a switch box that contains a finite number of switches. The network is invariant, but each switch can be in one of two positions, on or off. Unless the switches are set, nothing happens. But when the switches are set in one of the permissible ways, the system functions, yielding the entire array of interpretations for linguistic expressions. A slight change in switch settings can yield complex and varied phenomenal consequences as its effects filter through the network...To acquire a language, the child's mind must determine how the switches are set.... (Chomsky, 1988c:68).

Research within a UG paradigm attempts to discover the principles and parameters which capture the essential properties of all existing and possible natural languages. Although, apriori there might be an infinite number of different rule systems possible for a natural language, this work seeks to discover a finite set of principles and parameters which can characterize all possible language variation.

The principles and parameters theory proposes a very strong theory of L1 acquisition. As we have seen, the child is innately or biologically programmed to attend to certain aspects of possible language variation in the language data to which she is exposed, i.e., to certain dimensions of language variation, viz., a finite set of parameters. She sets the value of these dimensions of language organization when she is exposed to the relevant language data, and on the basis of doing so, a number of different facts of language organization can be derived deductively.

To briefly summarize, the essential claim of the theory of UG is that it constrains the language learner's hypotheses about which dimensions of language variation are significant in possible grammars for a language. It constrains these hypotheses by providing restricted, preferably binary, possible values for dimensions of variation, and as a result of choosing a particular value, UG provides multiple deductive consequences for grammar construction. Note that this theory says nothing about proficiency levels to be attained, a point which will be returned to later in this paper.

Two general ways to conceptualize a theory of UG for adult L2 acquisition

Given UG as an account of at least the L1 process, there are several ways in which one might want to consider the role of this theory in the adult L2 acquisition process. I will consider two current proposals here (See Flynn & Manuel, 1991; Flynn, Martohardjono & O'Neil, in preparation, for an extended discussion of other possibilities); these two possibilities differ both theoretically and empirically.

Possibility one: Fixed UG

Under the first approach, which will be called a FIXED UG, UG plays little or no role in the adult L2 acquisition process. Within this context, while UG in its entirety may inform and constrain child L1 acquisition, it is unavailable to the adult in this form. That is, while the child at the initial state may have available to her the entire set of options provided by a theory of UG, the adult L2 learner will either not have any of these options or only a very limited set available. Consider two representative scenarios: Schachter (1988, 1990) and Clahsen and Muysken (1989). In the case of Schachter, as outlined in 2, if some instantiation of a parameter is necessary for the acquisition of a new target L2 and it is not incorporated in the learner's L1 (i.e, not chosen), then this value will not be available to the adult.[5] With respect to UG, if the adult L2 learner only has available to her an L1 instantiated UG, then this suggests that the adult L2 acquisition is not constrained by UG in the same manner as is child L1 acquisition.

(2) Window of Opportunity Hypothesis (Schachter 1988):

> If there occur windows of opportunity associated with the maturation of the principles of UG, and if exposure to the second language does not occur until all such opportunities have passed, then all that remains as part of the knowledge state of an adult native speaker of a language is a language-specific instantiation of UG, that of the first language. UG in its entirety will not be available as a knowledge source for the adult acquisition of a second language. **Only a language-specific instantiation of it will**

> **be** (Schachter, 1988:13). (Emphasis mine) If, however, it turns out that in the acquisition of the target some instantiation of principle P is necessary and P is not incorporated into the learner's L1, the learner will have no language-internal knowledge to guide him/her in the development of P. Therefore, completeness with regard to the acquisition of the target language will not be possible (13-14).

As shown in (3), Clahsen and Muysken (1989) similarly argue that only an L1 instantiated UG is available to the adult L2 learner.

(3) Clahsen and Muysken's Position (1989):

> According to our view, the observed differences between L1 and L2 learning can be explained by assuming that child L1 acquisition falls under the parameter theory of language development, whereas the acquisition strategies used by adults in L2 development may be defined in terms of principles of information processing and general problem solving (1989:23). The basic difference, in our view, between child and adult language development is that children have direct access to UG, whereas adults only have access to UG as it is mediated through their mature L1 grammar. Thus, if German- or French-speaking adults are asked to give a grammaticality judgement of an English test sentence, **they can only fall back on UG principles in so far as these have instantiations in the speakers' own language** (1989: 26). (Emphasis mine) While both Schachter's and Clahsen and Muysken's approaches appeal to a theory of UG, they do so in a manner that focusses on UG outcomes based on the L1 acquisition process alone; the essential language faculty hypothesized for L1 acquisition is non-operative in the same form for the adult L2 learner.

Within these perspectives, UG as it is available to a child L1 learner does not constrain the adult L2 learner's hypotheses by providing restricted binary options about which dimensions of language are significant in possible grammars. These choices are restricted by UG only in the sense that the L1 has chosen certain UG options and not others. The primitives within this system are not really principles and parameters of UG but principles and parameters of a particular L1 grammar. Thus, by definition within this approach, L2 grammar construction will differ significantly from L1 grammar construction.

Possibility two: Dynamic UG

A second alternative perspective, which is very different from those considered above, takes as primitives all the principles and parameters delineated by a theory of UG in the L2 acquisition process. In general, such a position claims essentially that UG rather than the learner's L1 restricts the options available to the adult L2 learner. Within this framework, a parameter-setting model can be applied to the adult L2 acquisition in that, as in child L1 acquisition, principles and parameters of UG constrain the language learner's hypotheses about which dimensions of language variation are significant in possible grammars for language. Recall that UG, as outlined in (1), constrains these hypotheses by providing restricted (preferably binary) possible values for these dimensions of variation, and it provides multiple deductive consequences for grammar construction. Within this context, in contrast to Schachter's and Clahsen & Muysken's positions, the adult L2 learner is able to assign new values to parameters where the L1 and the L2 do not match. And, they do so in a manner evidenced in child L1 acquisition.

Initial development of this approach builds upon two already observed phenomena in the literature (see discussion in Flynn 1983; 1987): 1) Developmentally, many observed patterns of acquisition in adult L2 acquisition correspond to those chronicled for child L1 acquisition and, 2) the acquisition of a new target language is not primarily driven by the properties of the L1 grammar.

This approach incorporates the role of the L1 in the adult L2 acquisition process although in a manner that differs in certain critical ways from that envisaged within the FIXED approach. The DYNAMIC approach acknowledges that the adult L2 learner does not start with a clean slate i.e., the learner does not start at an initial state zero (S_0) with all parameters unset. It also argues that UG in its entirety is still available to the adult in contrast to the FIXED approach. UG continues to provide the adult with the full range of restricted binary options about dimensions of language variation in all possible languages, not just about those in the learner's L1. UG does not have a critical period wherein after a certain period of time it becomes unavailable or is altered in some way in the adult L2 acquisition process. The DYNAMIC position argues that the learner is able to assign new values to parameters where they differ between the L1 and the L2. And, the L2 learner accomplishes this in a manner comparable to that observed in child L1 acquisition. However, where the L1 and L2 match in parametric values, the adult learner can access this value and use it to guide her in the acquisition of the new target language. That is, there is no duplication of structure with respect to parametric values. In this case, learners do not assign the same value twice to a parameter as there is no need to do so. In the case in which the L1 and L2 differ in parametric values, the learner must and does assign a new value to the parameter. While in both cases, the developmental trajectory is sanctioned by a theory of UG, the two patterns may differ. Where the L1 and L2 match in parameter settings, acquisition is "facilitated;" where they do not match, acquisition is "disrupted" when compared to the case in which the L1 and L2 match (see discussion in Flynn 1987; Flynn 1988a).

Such a model does not deny that ostensible differences exist between child L1 and adult L2 acquisition. However, the DYNAMIC approach does not assume UG to be a proficiency model as is often argued (e.g., Bley-Vroman 1990). That is, the principal role of UG is to constrain the learner's hypothesis space. Explanations of child L1 and adult L2 acquisition differences need to be explained in terms of the complex interactions of the biologically endowed faculty for language and other extra-linguistic factors as argued elsewhere (Flynn and Manuel 1991; Flynn and Martohardjono 1990, 1991).

In short, the DYNAMIC approach assumes that the adult L2 learner, as the child L1 learner, constructs a grammar of the new target language constrained by principles and parameters of UG. Within this context, parameter-resetting or "new assignment" is possible.

General Empirical Predictions of the FIXED and DYNAMIC Models

Predictions for both the FIXED and DYNAMIC versions vary considerably: The FIXED model would predict no evidence of grammar construction in the manner observed in child L1 acquisition as all that is available to the adult L2 learner is an L1 instantiated UG along with more general problem solving strategies. Within this framework, rules that have already been learned in some sense are available to the learner but the ability to construct new rules under the constraint of a theory of UG is not. To accomplish this new learning, the learner would have to apply structure independent learning strategies to the acquisition of structures not licensed by a grammatical principle that matches in both the L1 and the L2. For example, a Japanese speaker would have to learn that English, in contrast to Japanese, is a head-initial language through some general problem solving strategy — however this might be accomplished. In addition, we would predict that errors made by learners acquiring new structures would also reflect a lack of the application of structure dependent hypotheses. Moreover, the acquisition of new structures would not match that for the L1 acquisition of these same forms. In short, L2 acquisition of structures not licensed by a grammatical principle that matches in both the L1 and the L2 should reflect some general problem solving strategy rather than being guided by principles and parameters of a theory of UG.

Alternatively, if the task of the adult L2 learner were to construct a theory of grammar for the new target language, and if the structures to be acquired were found to contrast with the grammar of the new target language, the DYNAMIC model would argue that the adult L2 learner could access those principles and parameters not available to her from the L1 in the construction of the L2 grammar. Within this context, the adult as does the child constructs a theory of grammar for the new target language under the constraint of principles an parameters of UG. In acquisition, we would expect to find evidence that L2 learners' hypotheses are structure dependent and that the nature of these constraints is provided by a theory of UG not by the L1 instantiations alone. Errors would systematically reflect the role of grammatical principles in acquisition and developmental patterns should correspond to those observed in child L1 acquisition in some fundamental way.

In order to test these general hypotheses, a sample set of empirical L2 acquisition data will be considered in order to see how explanatory each version is.

Experimental Data

In this section of the paper, a small set of results from two experimental studies will be summarized. To anticipate, results indicate that the adult L2 learner solves problems of complex sentence formation in a manner evidenced in L1 acquisition. At the same time, the results indicate a subtle interaction of the learner's L1 knowledge base in this acquisition process. These results are argued to provide important evidence for the direct role of a biologically specified program for language, essentially a parameter-setting model of UG in the adult L2 acquisition process.

Hypotheses

The general hypotheses to be tested in this paper are the following: If the adult L2 learner has no direct access to UG and only has access to an L1 instantiated UG as dictated by the FIXED approach, we would expect 1) no evidence to suggest that the learners are constructing a theory of grammar and, 2) errors made by the learners to reflect this lack of structural analysis.

If on the other hand, the adult L2 learner has direct access to UG and not just the L1 grammar, we might expect regardless of the match or mismatch of grammatical properties between the L1 and the L2 1) evidence that adult L2 learners are constructing a theory of grammar; specifically, the hypotheses entertained by the learners are constrained by a theory of UG and, 2) errors made by the learners would reflect structure dependent analyses.

Research Design

To test these general hypotheses, the L2 acquisition of English by adult Japanese speakers was empirically investigated. The basic facts about Japanese are well known as shown in 8. English is an SVO language and Japanese is an SOV language. In addition, English is a head-initial language — heads precede their complements and Japanese is a head-final language — complements precede their heads (Kuno, 1973).

(4) BASIC LINGUISTIC FACTS:

a. WORD ORDER:
ENGLISH: SVO
The doctor criticized the professor.
JAPANESE: SOV
Isha- wa kyoju- o hihanshita.
Doctor-topic professor-acc. criticized.
"The doctor criticized the professor".

b. HEAD-DIRECTION
ENGLISH: HEAD-INITIAL
The doctor who criticized the professor entered the room.
JAPANESE: HEAD-FINAL

Kyoju-	*o*	*hihanshita*	*isha-* *wa*	*heya-ni*	*haitta.*
Professor-acc.		criticized	doctor-topic	room-loc	entered

"The doctor who criticized the professor entered the room".

Results to be reported here derive from two larger studies investigating several other first language groups at several stages of English development (Flynn 1987; Flynn, Lardiere, and Babyonyshev 1989). The focus of this paper is on the Japanese speakers alone.

Prior to the actual experimental testing, these learners were placed into an ESL proficiency level group based on their results from the listening comprehension and grammar test from the Placement Test from the University of Michigan. Results from each of these sub-tests were identical for each speaker allowing us to make an ESL placement based on the combined score.

The subjects used for Study 1 are shown in (5) as well as those from study 2.

(5) JAPANESE SUBJECTS:
STUDY 1 (Flynn 1987):
OVERALL ESL LEVEL PLACEMENT

	#	SCORE (0-50)
LOW	7	20.0
MID	25	31.0
HIGH	21	42.0

STUDY 2 (Flynn, Lardiere, and Babyonyshev 1989):

	#	SCORE (0-50)
LOW	1	15.0
MID	5	31.0
HIGH	20	44.0

This paper will focus on the results of the High ESL proficiency group from each study; although the results for all three groups will be reported for Study 1.[6] Speakers from Test 1 were tested on the acquisition of complex subordinate sentence structures. Speakers from Test 2 were tested on coordinate sentence structures.[7]

Experimental Task

These learners were tested in their elicited imitation of sentences shown in (6). In an elicited imitation task, a learner is given a series of randomized sentences which she is then asked to repeat one by one after the experimenter. The basic assumption underlying such a task is that the learner must both comprehend and structurally analyze the sentence in order to provide an imitation. The actual utterance given by the learner thus provides us with some measure of the level of the learner's developing linguistic competence (see discussion in Flynn 1986; Lust, Chien and Flynn 1987).

Experimental Sentences

The learners were tested on essentially two types of sentences: coordinate and subordinate sentences. The coordinate sentence types tested involved both null and pronoun anaphors, a null anaphor in (6a) and a pronoun anaphor in (6b). In addition, both of these sentences involved forward anaphora structures. That is, the antecedent preceded the anaphors in both of the sentences. The subordinate sentences in (6c) and (10d) involved pre-posed adverbial subordinate clauses. In addition, the sentence in (6d) involved forward pronoun anaphora. Both of the pre-posed sentence structures, as already noted above, are very productive structures in Japanese.

(6) EXAMPLES OF STIMULUS SENTENCES: Coordinate Clauses:
a. TYPE I: Forward null anaphora
The doctor criticized the professor and entered the room.
b. TYPE II: Forward pronoun anaphora
The boss informed the lawyer and he studied the notebook.
Subordinate Clauses:
c. TYPE III: Pre-posed subordinate clause
When the man dropped the television the doctor called the child.
d. TYPE IV: Pre-posed subordinate clause/forward pronoun anaphora
When the professor opened the package, he answered the man.

The sentences were equalized in terms of number of syllables; they were also designed to be pragmatically neutral. In addition, all speakers were familiar with the lexical items before testing as well as with the experimental tasks.

Results

Results on amount correct for these sentences are shown in (7) and (8).

(7) COORDINATE CLAUSE RESULTS:
(SENTENCES 6A AND B)
MEAN AMOUNT CORRECT
(SCORE RANGE: 0-3)

	TYPE I: NULL	TYPE II: PRONOUN
HIGH	.55	.65

(8) SUBORDINATE CLAUSES:(SENTENCES 6C AND D)
MEAN AMOUNT CORRECT
(SCORE RANGE 0-3)

	TYPE III: NO ANAPHORA	TYPE IV: PRONOUN
LOW	.00	.00
MID	.24	.16
HIGH	.38	.95
OVERALL	.21	.37

Subsequent analyses of the errors made by the speakers in imitation of these sentences indicate the speakers converted coordinate sentences in (6) to subordinate structures. The per cent of this error is shown in (9). Examples are given in (10). Many of these conversions, especially for the null anaphora structures, were to post-posed infinitival clauses (Null: 43% of errors; Pronoun: 19% of errors). It is important to note that speakers converted coordinate sentences to subordinate sentences only when they involved anaphora. Results of other coordinate sentences not involving anaphora did not exemplify this high rate of conversion to subordination (see Flynn, Lardiere, and Babyonyshev 1989).

(9) ERROR ANALYSES CONVERSION OF COORDINATE SENTENCES TO SUBORDINATE SENTENCES
% OF ALL ERRORS

	TYPE I: NULL	TYPE II: PRONOUN
HIGH	62%	53%

(10) EXAMPLES OF ERRORS:

a. STIMULUS: The owner introduced the actor and prepared the breakfast.
RESPONSE: The owner introduced the actor to prepare the breakfast.

b. STIMULUS: The student criticized the engineer and he dropped the plans.
RESPONSE: The student criticize the engineer to drop the plans.

In addition, the speakers converted the subordinate sentence structures (Types III and IV) to coordinate sentence structures with identical NPs in subject position to a high degree. It is important to note that the speakers convert sentences with pre-posed clauses and forward anaphora (Type IV sentences) to coordinate sentences much more than they do subordinate sentences that do not involve forward anaphora (Type III sentences). In fact this accounted for the highest single error category for these Type IV sentence structures. This is shown in (11). Examples of the errors are shown in (12).

(11) ERROR ANALYSES:
CONVERSION OF SUBORDINATE SENTENCES TO COORDINATE SENTENCES

% OF ALL ERRORS

	TYPE III: NO ANAPHORA	TYPE IV: PRONOUN
LOW	19%	2%
MID	33%	34%
HIGH	35%	45%
OVERALL	32%	27%

(12) EXAMPLES OF ERRORS:

a. STIMULUS: When the worker called the owner when the engineer finished the plans.
RESPONSE: Worker called the owner and worker finished the plans.

b. STIMULUS: When the doctor received the results, he called the gentleman.
RESPONSE: The doctor received the results and the doctor called the gentleman.

Results Considered within a FIXED Approach

Overall, in contrast to our predictions for the FIXED approach, we did not find evidence for the application of general problem solving strategies in the acquisition of the structures tested. In addition, the results of the error analyses given in 9-12 above are not predicted by such a model. First, the FIXED approach would have predicted errors to be astructural, perhaps primarily lexical consistent with the fact that the adult L2 learners may, for example, attempt to translate item by item from the L1 to the L2 or apply some other general inductive problem solving strategy. Second, such an approach does not predict the systematic conversion of coordinate structures to subordinate ones or the conversion of subordinate to coordinate structures. These results, as will be discussed in more detail below, suggest the development of a unified theory of grammar for English and the fact that L2 learners are sensitive to specific grammatical configurations. Under the FIXED approach, the learner would not entertain any general theory of grammar for the new target language. In short, predictions for the FIXED approach remain unsupported.

Results Considered within a DYNAMIC Approach

The results reported in this paper force us to abandon a FIXED approach as an explanatory model of the adult L2 acquisition process and to consider a DYNAMIC approach explanation for the results.

First, the DYNAMIC approach predicted evidence that adult L2 learners could access principles and parameters not available in the L1 grammar. Recall that Japanese is principally a head-final language and English is principally a head-initial language yet evidence emerged which strongly suggests the fact that adult Japanese speakers are able to assign a new parametric value to the head-direction parameter in the acquisition of English and are not forced to acquire head-initial structures through some other nonlinguistic means.

Second, the results, along with the error analyses, also indicated that the learners were constructing a theory of English grammar. The learners demonstrated distinct sensitivities to particular structural configurations. For example, the learners did not treat all of the sentence structures comparably. They did not make the same errors on all structures which would have been predicted by a general problem solving approach to L2 acquisition. In the case at hand, the speakers distinguished between coordinate and subordinate structures; they also distinguished between sentences with no anaphora and those with anaphora, and they distinguished between null and pronoun anaphora. To summarize:

1. Empirical evidence that the adult learners are working out the grammar of English thus suggesting the continued role of UG in its entirety in the adult L2 acquisition process.
2. Results indicate the role of systematic, constrained hypotheses operative in the adult L2 acquisition process. This is evident when we consider the relationship evidenced in the data between coordination and subordination in the learner's hypotheses.

Thus, the DYNAMIC approach does provide us with the right set of predictions for the data reported here. Let us consider in more detail how such a model accounts for these data.

Detailed Account of the Data within a DYNAMIC Framework

More specifically, the DYNAMIC approach understands Japanese speakers' emerging grammars in terms of "resetting" of certain parametric values responsible for differences between the two languages within a theory of Universal Grammar.

First, I argue that the results reported here reflect the interdependence of L2 learners theories of anaphora and sentence configurations such as c-command — a complex structural relation that holds between constituents and one that plays an important role in a number of areas of syntax and semantics, namely in the proper description of anaphora relations.

Specifically, adult L2 learners develop theories of anaphora in close coherence with the preferred head-complement structure for the language they are learning — in this case, English as a head-initial language as shown in (4). L2 learners as do children learning L1s want and need to calibrate anaphora direction with the head-direction of the target language they are learning (see review in Lust 1986). To do this, they need such a structural configuration to help them set up their incipient hypotheses about anaphora as anaphora in the adult grammar crucially relies upon abstract structural configurations. In the case described in this paper, adult Japanese speakers want sentences in English to reflect a head-initial configuration; that is, they want complements to follow their heads and they want the anaphora direction to be in a forward direction. They want the antecedents to precede the anaphors in accordance with the head-initial configuration of English.

Since Japanese is a head-final language, these learners must revise their hypotheses about head-complementation in order to cohere with the structural facts about English. The results isolated here provide important new evidence with respect to attempts to insuring an anaphoric interpretation that is structurally consistent with their emerging theories of the head-complement structure of English.

When coordinate structures involve forward anaphora as in 16a&b, the Japanese learners converted these sentences to post-posed subordinate infinitival structures in closer accord with the head-initial configuration of English. That is, the main clause serves as a head followed by a complement in accord with the head-initial structure of English. At the same time, the learners want the anaphora to be structurally bound. Thus, they convert these structures to control-like configurations as exemplified in the infinitival clauses. In so doing, L2 learners ensure establishing the correct dominance relations necessary to interpret the anaphora in these sentences.

At the same time, and here the argumentation becomes a bit more subtle, when subordinate sentences such as in 6c&d do not involve anaphora, and when they do not involve true complements but adjuncts such as adverbial subordinate clauses, and when this entire structural configuration does not match the head-initial configuration of English, although they do match Japanese extensionally, these learners must and do make the following changes in accord with their developing theory of English grammar. First, they convert these adjunct clauses to a coordinate sentence structure — one in which neither sentence is an adjunct to the other. Such a conversion seems to be a syntactically necessary operation prior to the learner's ability to deal with one clause later as a complement.

Second, these coordinate sentences also involve a primitive form of bound anaphora. That is, the learners give us two identical NPs in subject position of each clause. The second NP can be reduced which would result in an antecedent preceding a null anaphor, essentially a forward anaphora relation.

Results from sentence (6d) (pre-posed clause and forward pronoun anaphora) provide additional evidence that learner's hypotheses about anaphora and head-complement configurations are tightly linked. When subordinate adjunct clauses involve forward anaphora and a structure that is in disaccord with the preferred head-complement structure for the L2 they are learning, learners also reduce these structures to coordinate sentences that involve forward anaphora. These results suggest that forward anaphora alone is not sufficient for these learners. They need forward anaphora in a true head-complement configuration in order to successfully process these sentences.

To conclude, results indicate a very complex picture for adult L2 acquisition, one that in many ways reflects deep deductive processes of learning evidenced in child L1 learning. Regardless of the L1 extensional facts available to a learner, if they do not cohere at deep levels of grammar construction with the L2, the learner will reconstruct a grammar of the new target language in accord with the underlying properties of the target L2 grammar. Within such a context, predictions made by FIXED type L2 acquisition theories will continue to fail to yield and capture the correct insights involved in the adult L2 acquisition process.

Within this context, linguistic theory plays a significant role for L2 acquisition. It specifies which dimensions of language variation learners will attend to and it provides the set of hypotheses learners will entertain about the target language grammar. It is important to notice what a theory of UG does not do, however; it does not explain lack of completeness or differences that emerge between children and adults in terms of attained proficiency. As discussed above, such explanations must derive from an understanding of the biologically endowed faculty for language in interaction with other domains of cognition (Flynn & Manuel, 1991; Flynn, Martohardjono & O'Neil, in preparation).

L2 Acquisition as a Constraint on Linguistic Theory

Within this context, a DYNAMIC model of adult L2 acquisition can constrain a theory of grammar by providing evidence about which dimensions of language are subject to variation precisely because L2 learning involves experience and acquisition demands isolating anew those properties of the L2 grammar that might be in variation with the L1. In addition, as recently argued by Chomsky (1988a,b), studies of adult L2 acquisition are unique in that they inform linguistic theory concerning the nature of end-states and steady-states. Essentially, adult L2 acquisition results challenge traditional formulations of steady states as static entities (Chomsky, 1988a,b).

L2 acquisition results also provide evidence for the distinction between variant and invariant principles and provide evidence with respect to the psychological reality of such a distinction. In addition, results of L2 acquisition contribute to a full elucidation of concepts concerning development especially with respect to such debates of continuity vs. maturation. Given the uniqueness of the adult with respect to advanced cognitive development and linguistic experience, the study of the adult L2 acquisition process can inform linguistic theory in ways not provided by the study of L1 acquisition alone.

Conclusion

To conclude, given the current rapid rate of progress in both linguistic theory and adult L2 acquisition, continued investigation will make more precise the exact nature of the interplay between these two domains and in this way contribute to the entire domain of cognitive science and elevate the study of L2 acquisition to the empirical and theoretical status it rightfully deserves.

Notes

1. The author wishes to thank the editor of this volume and the participants at the conference for their insightful comments, suggestions and questions concerning the issues raised in this paper. The author would also like to thank one anonymous reviewer for useful comments for revision.
2. While it might be logically possible that theoretical linguistics has little or nothing to say about L2 learning, *a priori* one cannot simply assume this position as is often done.
3. This does not rule out the subtle role of the L1 in L2 acquisition as we will see later in this paper.
4. In this paper, the term "second language learning" is meant to refer to both naturalistic L2 learning and classroom foreign language learning. Both enterprises are concerned with individuals who come to "know" or master a new target language. Thus, for the purposes of this paper, we will treat them synonymously (see related discussion in Rutherford 1987).

In addition, this paper is primarily concerned with the adult L2 learning process essentially because most recent investigations of L2 acquisition have focused on this population. While I would like to believe that the conclusions reached here with respect to adults also extend to child L2 learning, without more empirical evidence, generalizations of this form are premature.

5. Schachter's proposal actually consists of two contingent parts: one, the postulation of a critical period for parameter settings, and two, the nature of the acquisition process after the critical period stage. This paper focusses on the second part of Schachter's claims. For a more detailed discussion of part two, see Flynn and Manuel (1991) and Flynn, Martohardjono and O'Neil (in preparation) and Martohardjono and Gair (this volume).

6. The data from Study 2 for the Low and Mid proficiency groups, while matching the trends isolated for the High group is yet too scant to be reliably reported. An extended set of results with more speakers at these two levels will be reported in Flynn, Lardiere and Babyonshev (in preparation).

7. The profiles of the Japanese speakers in both Study 1 and 2 were comparable. For the purposes of this paper, speakers at the High level were from the same socio-economic backgrounds (all were graduate students or professionals); the number of years of ESL study matched, and most importantly, both groups were comparable in terms of their ESL proficiency levels as measured by the Michigan Test. This comparability between the two groups allows us to assume that each group tested is representative of their group. this in turn allows us to combine the results from the two studies.

8. This difference in the amount of conversion of the null and pronoun anaphor to infinitival sentence structures suggests that the speakers distinguish the two types of anaphors in these structures at some level. For a more extended discussion see Flynn, Lardiere and Babyonshev (1989).

9. The low percent of conversion to coordination at the Low level for Type IV sentences reflects the fact in contrast to the errors made on the Type III sentences that the speakers were unable to maintain the requisite two clause structure necessary for such an error to be tabulated. For an extended discussion of this result see Flynn and Manuel (1991).

10. More technically, we can understand c-command in the following way: "X c-commands Y iff the first branching node dominating X domiantes Y, and X does not dominate Y, nor Y dominate X." For more detailed discussion see e.g. Chomsky (1986).

11. One anonymous reviewer argued that there is an alternative explanation for the results presented in this paper. However, the reviewer failed to develop such an explanation in any way. thus, in the face of no such counterproposal, I am unable to address the questions this reviewer might have had.

References

Bley-Vroman, R. 1989. "What is the Logical Problem of Foreign Language Learning?" *Linguistic Perspectives on Second Language Acquisition* ed. by S. Gass and J. Schachter, 41-68. Cambridge: Cambridge University Press.

Chomsky, N. 1986a. *Barriers*. Cambridge, MA: MIT Press.

Chomsky, N. 1986b. *Knowledge of Language: Its Nature, Origin, and Use*. New York: Praeger Publishers.

Chomsky, N. 1988a. "Some Notes on Economy of Derivation and Representation". Ms. MIT.

Chomsky, N. 1988b. "Linguistics and Adjacent Fields: The State of the Art." Ms. MIT.

Chomsky, N. 1988c. *Language and Problems of Knowledge: The Managua Lectures*. Cambridge, MA. MIT Press.

Clahsen, H. and P. Muysken. 1989. "The UG Paradox in L2 Acquisition." *Second Language Research* 5.1-19.

Flynn, S. 1983. *A Study of the Effects of Principal Branching Direction in Second Language Acquisition: The Generalization of a Parameter of Universal Grammar from First to Second Language Acquisition*. Ph.D Diss. Cornell University.

Flynn, S. 1986. "Comprehension vs. Production." *Studies in Second Language Acquisition* 8.17-46.

Flynn, S. 1987. *A Parameter-Setting Model of L2 Acquisition: Experimental Studies in Anaphora*. Dordrecht: Reidel.

Flynn, S. 1988a. "Nature of Development in L2 Learning and Implications for Theories of Language Acquisition in General." Flynn and O'Neil 1988.76-89.

Flynn, S. 1988b. "Linguistic Theory and Foreign Language Learning and Teaching." Paper presented at the National Foreign Language Center Conference, Bellagio, Italy. To appear in the conference proceedings.

Flynn, S. and W. O'Neil, eds. 1988. *Linguistic Theory in Second Language Acquisition*. Dordrecht: Kluwer Academic Publishers.

Flynn, S. and S. Manuel. 1991. "Age Dependent Effects in Adult L2 Learning: An Examination of Critical Period Hypotheses." Paper presented at Second Language Research Forum 1989, Los Angeles. To appear in *Point Counterpoint: Universal Grammar in the Second Language* ed. by L. Eubank. 117-146.

Flynn, S., D. Lardiere, and M. Babyonyshev. 1989. "Coordination vs. Subordination in Adult L2 Acquisition of English Anaphora." Paper presented at the International Linguistics Association, April, 1989. Revised extended version in preparation.

Flynn, S. and G. Martohardjono. 1990. "Critical Periods in L2 Acquisition." Paper presented at the meeting of International Association of Applied Linguistics, Thessoloniki, Greece.

Flynn, S. and G. Martohardjono. 1991. "How Critical Is Age in Adult L2 Learning." Paper presented at American Association for the Advancement of Science Annual Meeting, Washington, D.C. Extended version in preparation.

Flynn, S., G. Martohardjono and W. O'Neil. In preparation. "UG in Adult L2 Acquisition: A Clarification of the Issues."

Fodor, G., M. Garrett and T. Bever. 1974. *The Psychology of Language: An Introduction to Psycholiguistics and Generative Grammar*. New York: McGraw Hill.

Kuno, Susumo. 1973. *The Structure of the Japanese Language*. Cambridge, MA: MIT Press.

Lust, B. 1986. "Introduction." *Studies in the Acquisition of Anaphora, Vol.1: Defining the Constraints*. ed. by B. Lust, 6-103. Dordrecht: D. Reidel Publishing Company.

Lust, Barbara, Yu Chin Chien and Suzanne Flynn. 1987. "What Children Know: Methods for the Study of First Language Acquisition." *Studies in the Acquisition of Anaphora, Volume 2: Applying the Constraints* ed. by B. Lust, 271-356. Dordrecht: D. Reidel Publishing Company.

Martohardjono, G. and J. Gair. 1989. "Apparent Inaccessibility in SLA: Misapplied Principles or Principled Misapplications?" This Volume.

Schachter, J. 1990. "On the Issue of Completeness in Second Language Acquisition." *Second Language Research* 6.93-124.

Watt, W. 1970. "On Two Hypotheses Concerning Psycholinguistics." *Cognition and the Development of Language*. ed. by J. Hayes, 137-220. New York: Wiley.

Metrical Phonology and the Acquisition of L2 Stress[1]

John Archibald
The University of Calgary

Domain of Inquiry

Most parameter-related research has taken place in the area of syntax. Flynn (1987) looked at the head-initial/head-final parameter; Phinney (1987) looked at pro-drop; White (1985) looked at subjacency; etc. There has been little done in the area of phonology with the notable exception of Dresher and Kaye 1990 (see also Ioup and Weinberger 1987 and Mairs 1989).

The Acquisition of Stress Project

The study I shall be describing in this paper is part of a larger project known as the Acquisition of Stress Project (ASP). The ASP is designed to investigate the acquisition of English stress patterns by adult, non-native speakers of English. Specifically, the behaviour of learners from three different language types (with respect to stress) is being studied: Spanish, Hungarian, and Polish.

The ASP has four major objectives:

- To come to a better understanding of when the first language (L1) will transfer to the second language (L2).
- To collect some empirical evidence relevant to deductive theories of language acquisition.
- To investigate the pedagogic implications of this deductive view of language learning.
- To gather some data relevant to the Continuity Assumption in language acquisition research (cf. Pinker 1984).

Why Stress?

It makes sense to investigate stress within this framework for three main reasons:

- A well-developed theory of stress within a parametric framework exists — that is metrical phonology.
- It may help us to predict what linguistic features will be transferred from L1 to L2.
- Accentual systems can be studied in relative independence of other aspects of grammar.

English Stress

English verbs and unsuffixed adjectives exhibit some interesting properties. These words receive final stress if they end in a string of at least two consonants or a syllable having a long vowel, and otherwise penultimate stress (Hayes 1981). Examples are shown in (1).

(1) ro**bust**[2] **com**mon
o**vert** il**li**cit

Hayes' interpretation of this fact is that word-final consonants are extrametrical (invisible to stress assignment). This reflects the quantity-sensitive nature of English stress: branching rimes are stressed while non-branching rimes are not.

Many suffixed adjectives behave differently than unsuffixed ones, in that they follow the same pattern as regular nouns. Typically they are the ones that end with -al, -ous, -ant, -ent, and -ive, as shown in (2).

(2) mu**ni**cipal mag**na**nimous
sig**ni**ficant **in**nocent
primitive

Here we note that adjectival suffixes become extrametrical in final position. The exceptions to this rule are the suffixes -ic and -id which are almost always given penultimate stress, as if they were monomorphemic. Examples are given in (3).

(3) in**tre**pid eco**no**mic

One suffix that appears to be quantity insensitive is the -ate suffix which always places stress two syllables to its left, as in (4).

(4) **de**signate ar**ti**culate
confiscate **con**centrate

The Cycle

English stress applies cyclically. That is, it applies to the internal bracketed domains of derived words before applying to the word as a whole, as the examples in (5) show.

```
        3  4    1
(5)   [indent] ation from indent

         3    0   1
      [compensat] ion from compensate
```

(from in**dent**; from **com**pensate)

Spanish Stress

There is no such thing as an irregularly stressed verb form in Spanish (Harris 1983). Information regarding non-verb stress must be supplied in the lexicon; segmental representation and morphological characterization are necessary but not sufficient to determine word stress. However, stress placement is not totally free due to residual effects of the Latin stress rule (like English). Two points are of interest here:

- Stress must fall on one of the last three syllables of the word. Although a**ta**pama and ata**pa**ma are well-formed hypothetical words, ***a**tapama is not.
- Antepenultimate stress is impossible if the penult is a closed syllable. Hypothetical ata**pam**ba and atapam**ba** are well-formed but *a**ta**pamba is not (nor ***a**tapamba).

Although stress may appear on any of the last three syllables not all probabilities are equally likely. The following two generalizations are noted:

- Penultimate stress is unmarked in vowel final words:

  Unmarked: pis**to**la, per**di**da, sa**ba**na
  Marked: e**pis**tola, **per**dida, **sa**bana, Pana**ma**

- Final stress is unmarked in consonant-final words:

Unmarked: ci**vil**, mer**ced**, al**tar**
Marked: **mo**vil, **ces**ped, **am**bar

Stress assignment in Spanish is non-cyclic with the exception of two suffixes: -mente adverbs and the -ito diminutive.

The Study

This pilot study was designed to investigate a proposed parameter of quantity-sensitivity (cf. Dresher and Kaye 1990). I assigned two tasks to seven native speakers of Spanish. In the first task the subject was asked to read a list of fifty English words out loud into a tape recorder. Later I transcribed where each subject placed the stress on the word. The second task was a perception test in which the subjects listened to a native speaker pronounce each of the words twice from a tape. After a training session, their task was to mark which syllable they perceived the stress to be on. The perception task was conducted second in order that the production task not be influenced.

Why A Production Task?

Some of the research studies (e.g. White 1985) rely on grammaticality judgement tests in order to investigate the learners' parameter settings. Thus, the subjects' ability to perceive violations in the target language data is equated with their having acquired the L2 parameter setting. The study of stress seems particularly amenable to teasing apart production and perception variables. In this study, I hope to show that even though the learners are able to perceive the correct stress in the L2, their production may still be influenced by the L1. Therefore, we cannot infer actual parameter settings from perception data alone.

The Words

The following classes of words were presented to the subjects (with the words in random order):

Class 1. Anecdote, interface, kindergarten, undertow.
Since Spanish stress assignment does not allow antepenultimate stress when the penult is closed, we would predict that these words would be difficult for Spanish speakers if they are transferring their L1 metrical rules.

Class 2. Data, study, era, into, money.
The unmarked stress pattern for vowel-final words is penultimate. We would predict that these words would be produced correctly.

Class 3. Apply, construe, ago, supply, below.
Final stress is the marked stress pattern for vowel-final words. Thus, these words might be more difficult for Spanish speakers to produce.

Class 4. Explain, retrieve, afford, control.
Final stress is the unmarked pattern for Spanish consonant-final words. Thus, we would predict few problems with these words.

Class 5. Central, basis, reason, mountain, vowel, utmost.
Penultimate stress is the marked pattern for Spanish consonant-final words. Perhaps these words will cause problems for the Spanish speakers.

Class 6. Currently, secondary, stresslessness, relationship, frequency.
These derived forms were tested to see if the same constraint as in Class #1 applies to derived forms (for the most part Spanish stress assignment is non-cyclic.)

Class 7. Cannonball, overboard, undermine, sabertooth, basketball.
These words were tested in order to see if compounds exhibit the same constraint as in Class #1.

Class 8a. Robust, overt, collect.
English verbs and unsuffixed adjectives receive final stress if they end in a consonant cluster. It would be predicted that Spanish speakers would have difficulty with this.

Class 8b. Common, illicit.
English verbs and unsuffixed adjectives receive penultimate stress in other cases.

Class 9. Municipal, significant, magnanimous, innocent, primitive.
Many English adjectival suffixes are extrametrical. Spanish speakers may have difficulty acquiring this.

Class 10. Economic, intrepid.
The two exceptional suffixes are -ic and -id (which draw the stress to the immediately preceding syllable).

Class 11. Designate, confiscate, articulate, concentrate.
The -ate suffix in English is quantity-insensitive. The stress is always placed two syllables to the left of the suffix. It is predicted that Spanish speakers will have difficulty with this quantity-insensitivity.

The Results

First of all, let me say that we should only view this as a pilot study as there are only seven subjects. However, as each class of words has approximately five members, our sample size is not that bad.

Production versus Perception

The chart in (6) illustrates the breakdown of production versus perception errors:

(6) Total number of tokens (50 words X 7 subjects): 350
Production errors: 94 (27%)
Perception errors: 63 (18%)

While this is not as large a difference as might have been expected, I think it can be explained when we look at the individual results, shown in (7).

(7)

Subject #	% Production error	% Perception error
1	26%	4%
2	10%	1%
3	18%	3%
4	15%	0%
5	18%	20%
6	13%	21%
7	8%	16%

The first four subjects show a marked difference between their production and perception error rates. The final three subjects show, surprisingly I think, that they make more perception than production errors. Solely on the basis of the interview session, I would say that these students seemed to be lower in overall proficiency than the first four students, even though the number of production errors was about the same. Perhaps beginning students are less able to perceive differences in stress; they are still filtering the English through a Spanish sound system. The more advanced students are able to perceive the differences but are not yet able to put it into practice consistently.

Two Lexicons

Menn (1983) presents an interesting model which can be used to describe children's phonological knowledge. This is summarized in (8).

(8)

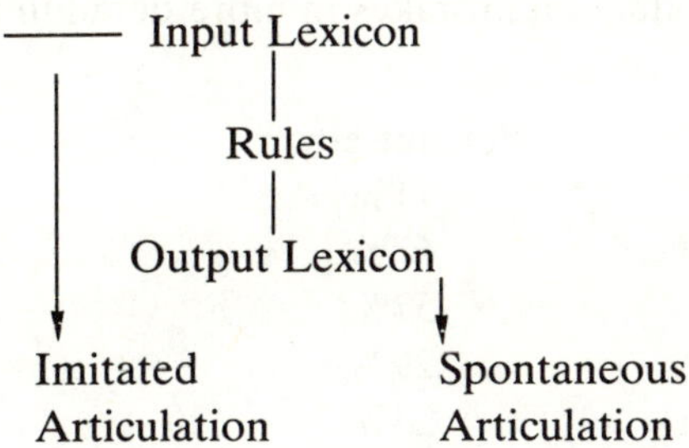

This two-lexicon model allows us to explain learners who are able to perceive distinctions that they are unable to make. The input lexicon stores a recognition form; the output lexicon stores a production form. Thus, if the learner, at a certain stage, is able to perceive which syllable is stressed in target speech but is unable to produce the word correctly, we would say there is a mismatch between the form stored in the input lexicon and the form stored in the output lexicon, as, for example, in (9).

(9) Input: **ba**by
|
Output: ba**by**

Note also the prediction that sometimes the output lexicon can be bypassed and a form uttered that comes directly from the input lexicon.

Menn's model might help us to explain the difference in behaviour of the students. The first four subjects have a fairly accurate input representation but their output representation is still influenced by L1 metrical structures. Subjects 5, 6, and 7, though, have still not developed an adequate input representation, so the production and perception forms are influenced by L1 and the error rates are more equal. Assuming that subjects 5, 6, and 7 are beginning students, these results support Menn's claim that the input representation is the first to normalize, with the output lexicon lagging behind.

It should also be noted that perception errors affected more words than production errors (36 versus 29) and that fewer people made mistakes on the same word. That is to say that in the production data there were fifteen words that three or more people made a mistake on. In the perception data, there were only five words that three or more people made a mistake on. Perhaps then, the production data is more reflective of the L1 interference.

Let us now look at the production mistakes in more detail in the chart in (10).

(10)

Class		Percent error
1	(heavy penult):	71%
8a	(final CC):	67%
10	(-ate suffix):	57%
11	(-ic and -id):	29%
9	([+ex] suffixes):	23%
7	(compounds):	20%
3	(marked V-final):	17%
5	(marked C-final):	17%
6	(derived forms):	14%
4	(unmarked C-final):	14%
2	(unmarked V-final):	0%
8b	(unmarked adj.):	0%

Generally speaking, this chart shows the kind of progression that we would expect to see. Class 1 words, which violate the Spanish stress assignment rules, are problematic. Class 8 words show that the subjects have not yet acquired the English constraint which gives final stress to words like robust and overt.[3] Class 10 words indicate that the Spanish speakers do have trouble with quantity-insensitive suffixes like -ate. They also have difficulty with adjectival suffixes whether they be extrametrical or fixed-stress giving. The subjects had problems with English compound stress too.

Considering the markedness factors, we note that there is some indication that production of marked forms may be slightly more difficult. Harris

(1983) who made these markedness claims does not give any information as to the frequencies of these phonological forms in Spanish. It is interesting to note, however, the radical difference in behaviour between Class 1 and Class 6 words shown in (11).

	Class 1	Class 6
(11)	Class 1	Class 6
	anecdote	currently
	interface	secondary
	kindergarten	stresslessness
	undertow	relationship
		frequency
	% errors: 71%	% errors: 14%

Both classes are examples of words which receive antepenultimate stress when the penult is closed, which violates Spanish stress-assignment rules. Class 6 words, though, seem to cause very few problems. No one made any mistakes on *stresslessness* or *relationship*; one person made a mistake on *currently*; and two people made mistakes on *secondary* and *frequency*. This would seem to indicate that the Spanish speakers have determined (at some level) that English stress assignment is cyclic.

Table 1 shows all the words with production errors and the number of subjects who erred.

Table 1. Production Mistakes Ranked

a**nec**dote (7)
robust (6)
de**sig**nate (6)
inter**face** (4)
in**ter**face (2)
construe (6)
moun**tain** (6)
overt (5)
confis**cate** (3)
con**fis**cate (1)
under**tow** (4)
concen**trate** (3)
con**cen**trate (1)
kinder**gar**ten (3)
articu**late** (3)
collect (3)
retrieve (3)
significant (3)

over**board** (2)
municipal (2)
intre**pid** (2)
economic (2)
secon**dary** (1)
se**con**dary (1)
fre**quen**cy (2)
can**non**ball (1)
cannon**ball** (1)
in**no**cent (1)
inno**cent** (1)
under**mine** (2)
cur**rent**ly (1)
afford (1)
magna**ni**mous (1)
saber**tooth** (1)

Quantity-sensitivity violations explain some of the most common mistakes: anecdote (7), robust (6), interface (6), overt (5), undertow (4), kindergarten (3), and collect (3).

Markedness violations are also explanatory. Several common mistakes resulted from the assignation of the unmarked stress pattern incorrectly: construe (6), mountain (6), concentrate (4), confiscate (4), and articulate (3).

These twelve words, then, account for 80% of the errors. Thus, quantity-sensitivity and markedness violations are definite sources of error.

Conclusion

The results of this study seem to indicate that Spanish speakers are transferring the metrical parameters of their L1 into the L2. The question is then: how will these parameters be reset?

I think that one of the most useful sources of information for the learner will be the mismatch between production and perception. Hyams (1987) talks of triggering data which is inconsistent with the current grammar and forces a resetting of a parameter. I think it is reasonable to assume that if the learner is not able to perceive native-speaker stress placement correctly, then this input will not act as triggering data. This seemed to be the case with the three lower level subjects in this study. However, once perception ability improves then some data will become available as triggering data due to the mismatch between perception and production.

I believe that this kind of study also has interesting implications for the idea that a single utterance will force the resetting of a parameter. This is obviously not the case in the above data. Often, performance variability is explained by referring to other cognitive processes involved in performance (Crain 1987). Yet, in this type of study of phonology I think it would be questionable to say that it involves the same degree of higher cognitive processes. And we have seen that there is quite a difference between the production and the perception.

Finally, I suggest that this study shows us that we must be wary of inferring parameter settings from perception results alone. The mismatch of production and perception may be crucial in making the triggering data available as intake to the learner. We must still address the question of what drives the change in the input representation. For example, could there be some sort of threshold or critical point at which the input representation will change? Right now we have no answers. However, the study of metrical parameters seems particularly well-suited to investigating many of the questions.

Notes

1. I would like to thank Elan Dresher, Susanne Carroll, Merrill Swain, and Birgit Harley for their comments on earlier drafts of this paper.
2. A syllable in bold face indicates a stressed syllable.
3. This is counter-evidence to Mairs' (1989) Marked Rime Hypothesis, as I understand it. For Spanish speakers to be getting these words wrong, they must be marking the whole coda as extrametrical. If only the final consonants are extrametrical, we would predict correct stress. For more on this, see Archibald, forthcoming.

References

Archibald, J. Forthcoming. "The Learnability of Metrical Parameters". To appear *International Review of Applied Linguistics*.

Crain, S. 1987. "How grammars help language learners." *University of Connecticut Working Papers in Linguistics*.

Dresher, E. and J. Kaye 1990. "A Computational Learning Model for Metrical Phonology". *Cognition* 34.137-195.

Flynn, S. 1987. *A Parameter Setting Model of Second Language Acquisition*. Dordrecht: D. Reidel Publishing Company.

Harris, J. 1983. *Syllable Structure and Stress in Spanish*. Cambridge, MA: MIT Press.

Hayes, B. 1981. *A Metrical Theory of Stress Rules*. Massachusetts Institute of Technology doctoral dissertation.

Hyams, N. 1987. "The theory of parameters and syntactic development." Roeper and Williams 1987.1-22.

Ioup, G. and S. Weinberger, eds. 1987. *Interlanguage Phonology*. Rowley, MA: Newbury House.

Mairs, Jane. 1989. "Stress Assignment in Interlanguage Phonology: An Analysis of the Stress System of Spanish Speakers Learning English". *Linguistic Perspectives on Second Language Acquisition* ed. by S. Gass and J. Schachter, 260-283. Cambridge: Cambridge University Press.

Menn, L. 1983. "Development of articulatory, phonetic, and phonological capabilities." *Language Production, volume 2* ed. by B. Butterworth. New York: Academic Press.

Phinney, M. 1987. "The pro-drop parameter in second language acquisition." Roeper & Williams 1987.221-238.

Pinker, S. 1984. *Language Learnability and Language Development*. Cambridge, MA: Harvard University Press.

Roeper, T. and E. Williams, eds. 1987. *Parameter Setting*. Dordrecht: D. Reidel Publishing Company.

White, L. 1985. "The acquisition of parameterized grammars: subjacency in second language acquisition." *Second Language Research* 1.1-17.

Phrasal Category Markedness and Second Language Acquisition

Mark Balhorn
University of Wisconsin-Madison

This paper is part of a long line of research that has sought to demonstrate the influence of markedness on first and second language acquisition. Some of the first studies in this vein were those of Klima and Bellugi (1966) and Brown, Cazden and Bellugi (1968), who, filled with enthusiasm over Chomsky's (1965, 1970) early grammars, thought they had found a good literal model of cognitive language processes. The assumption made was that this grammatical model could be used to determine the relative psycholinguistic complexity of one structure over another related one and that the one deemed less complex would be acquired before the other. Though the method of determining relative markedness changed with the evolution of the generative model, the assumption that markedness means psycholinguistic complexity continued to be utilized throughout the 1970's. This was true whether markedness was determined by the derivational complexity of the then current model, as in Dulay and Burt (1974) and Bresnan (1978), or whether it was determined by semantic notions of psycholinguistic complexity, such as number of semantic features, as in Clark (1973), or greater and lesser semantic opacity, as in Kellerman (1979).

Rutherford (1984) and later Zobl (1983) were the first to mention the circularity of defining markedness as psycholinguistic complexity. The question they raised is this: Is a structure marked because it is psycholinguistically difficult to process or is a structure rendered difficult to process by virtue of its markedness? The impossibility of answering this question led subsequent research to change its focus in three ways: First, a basis for establishing markedness empirically was sought for and located in studies of linguistic typology, such as those of Greenberg (1966) and Keenan and Comrie (1977). This approach has revealed frequencies and distributions of grammatical categories across languages of the world from which universal or near universal principles can be derived to account for the presence or absence of a particular structure in a particular language. Second, the formal, language specific descriptions of generative grammar are no longer expected to reveal the relative complexity of particular structures and an expected order of acquisition; instead, recent theories of generative grammar (Chomsky 1981; 1986) have attempted to establish a universal grammar (UG) composed of the abstract principles believed to underlie all human language. Since it is the settings of these parameterized principles that accounts for the variety of human languages, knowledge of the parametric settings of a particular language and what the settings entail elsewhere in the grammar, allow for the determination of a core grammar. Various structures can thus be determined as lying within the bounds of the core grammar or without (Van Reimsdijk and Williams 1986). Though those outside may be deemed marked and might therefore reveal themselves in acquisition data, not much can be said about the relative markedness or acquisition order of those inside. Finally, in the absence of supposed psycholinguistic processes, the late acquisition of marked constructions can be explained in terms of what Zobl (1983) calls "learnability", or what White (1982) refers to as a requirement for "positive evidence". This means that though language learners will produce unmarked constructions in spite of actual exposure to them, marked constructions will only enter the interlanguage of learners if there is positive evidence that such constructions, outside of the core grammar, exist in the target language.

This study is consistent with the first two research developments above in that it seeks to establish the markedness of a structure independently of any psycholinguistic assumptions, but it is dissimilar in that it does not attempt to discover chronological acquisition data that will illustrate the learnability principle of markedness. It is not that I doubt the existence at some level of such a principle; it is that I doubt any researcher can control for the linguistic exposure that may override this principle and bury it in even the most carefully collected data. As an example, let us briefly examine a study by Mazurkewich (1984, 1985) involving the acquisition of pied-piped movements vs. their counterpart movements which leave behind a stranded preposition, namely, unmarked, constructions such as (1).

(1) To whom [S were you speaking [PP____]]

and its marked counterpart, (2).

(2) Who [S were you speaking [PP to____]]

The latter construction is considered the marked one on three counts: First, it violates the subjacency principle of universal grammar (Van Reimsdijk and Williams 1986) whereby an element such as 'who' above normally cannot cross two bounding nodes, in this case PP and S. Additionally, preposition stranding such as that in the latter sentence above, is infrequent in the languages of the world while the former pied-piped construction is not. Finally, in implicational terms, although there are languages that have only pied-piping, as well as languages that have pied-piping and allow stranding, there are no languages that have only stranding constructions. Thus, stranding implies pied-piping, but not vice versa (White 1987).

In her study involving Inuit and Quebecois French school children who were learning English, Mazurkewich found that the French speakers tended to produce unmarked, pied-piped constructions while the Inuit speakers produced more marked, stranded constructions as well as double preposition constructions of the type in (3):

(3) To who [S were you speaking [PP to____]]

In discussing these results, she claimed that the French native speakers stranded fewer prepositions because they were not as far along in their acquisition of English as the Inuit were. The Inuit, "educated mainly in English after the third grade" (Mazurkewich 1985:25), had been exposed to marked constructions already and their production of double preposition constructions was evidence of an intermediate stage as they progressed from the unmarked to the marked. Although Mazurkewich later said that the Inuit results were "equivocal", she still maintained that the results from the French speakers supported the claim that "unmarked dative questions in an active context are acquired before marked ones" (Mazurkewich 1985:26).

However, even this is questionable. An equally adequate and much more plausible explanation of her results runs as follows: Given that Wh-movement with stranded prepositions is ubiquitous in all but the most formal styles of spoken English as well as most styles of written English, can either the Inuit or French group be shown not to have received positive evidence of the marked structure from the very first moment that they were exposed to English? As Mazurkewich states, limited preposition stranding is a feature of some Quebecois dialects, but not of standard French. Certainly, her French-speaking subjects are aware of this dialectal markedness and would not find this dialect feature appropriate in the French classroom.

Would it not seem likely that they might transfer this sociolinguistic markedness as regards stranded prepositions to the English classroom where one assumes her study was conducted? In addition, given the French speakers' sensitivity to the dialectal markedness of stranded prepositions in their own language, would they not be even more likely to pick up on the stylistical markedness of stranded prepositions in English, and hence think them inappropriate for the English classroom? Her French subjects, therefore, may well generate stranded prepositions when speaking English outside the classroom, and they may even have learned to strand prepositions in Wh-movements before they learned to pied-pipe them.

The reason for examining the Mazurkewich study is only to show that an effort to find patterns in acquistion of grammatical competence that square with characterizations of core grammar can be confounded by factors of language use and exposure, and to suggest that learners of English as a second language acquire not only grammatical competence, but other forms of language competence too.

English Genitives

This paper concerns the use of genitive constructions by native and nonnative speakers of English. In Table 1, are two columns of English genitive constructions. Column one contains the Genitive-Noun constructions in which the adjunct precedes the head, while the second column contains the Noun-Genitive counterpart construction in which the adjunct follows the head in a prepositional phrase. Notice that this is a broad definition of genitive, especially in regard to the preposed adjunct type. It includes both overtly marked genitives, such as 'tomorrow's forecast' as well as those containing bare adjuncts, such as the front stressed "law office" and the even stressed "speech security".

Table 1. Types of Genitive Construction

Genitive-Noun (GN)	Noun-Genitive (NG) or (N prep N)
tomorrow's forecast	forecast for tomorrow
law office	office of law
speech security	security at the speech

The first type of genitive, those marked with "s", were excluded from the study on the grounds that their productivity is limited when used with non-human head nouns. Furthermore, EFL students are often taught prescriptive guidelines in the use of genitive "s"; thus, their responses to genitives with "s" might reflect prior classroom instruction rather than markedness. The second type of genitive, that with fronted stress, exemplified here by "law office", is considered by most people to be a compound, not a genitive, and although there are many problems in drawing a strict or even general correlation between stress and compound status, such complications will be avoided in this study since only one out of the ten test constructions in this study carries fronted stress.[1] Therefore, the object of this study is even-stressed, noun-noun constructions in which the first noun is an adjunct modifying the following head noun and their noun-preposition-noun counterparts, in which the head noun is followed by a prepositional phrase, as in the pair "kitchen windows" vs. "windows in the kitchen".

Typological Markedness

The fact that English has both preposed and postposed genitives is odd in itself according to Hawkins (1982), since "most languages have only one". As for which one is the marked one, let us begin by examining the typology of the most common language types. Notice in Table 2 that English is a type 2 language in regard to main clause word order and adposition, but allows both types of genitive as well as the disharmonic order of noun and adjective. One might be tempted to say here that though English is a type 2 language, it is marked both in regard to adjective and genitive phrases; but Hawkins (1979) cautions against this conclusion. Unlike VSO languages and SOV languages, types 1 and 3 respectively, wherein the operators S and O are on the same side of V, English, as a type 2, SVO language has operators S and O on either side of the operand V. These opposing operators exert a kind of counterforce to the usual strict serialization of the respective adjunct and head ordering that is characteristic of VSO and SOV languages, and thus, SVO languages are more likely to diverge from their predominant head-adjunct serialization pattern. This can be seen in Table 3 regarding the frequency of type 2 SVO/Pr languages. Not only do the number of languages decrease as the incidence of prehead modification in the noun phrase increases, but there are 10 AN languages and only 2 GN

Table 2. Typological Markedness: Most Common Language Types

1. VSO/Pr/NG/NA	
2. SVO/Pr/NG/NA	(English: SVO/Pr/NG & GN/AN)
3. SOV/Po/GN/AN	
4. OSV/Po/GN/NA	
	(Comrie 1981:89)

Table 3. Frequencies of Type 2 SVO/Pr Languages

1. SVO & Pr & NA & NG	20 languages
2. SVO & Pr & AN & NG	8 languages
3. SVO & Pr & AN & GN	2 languages
	(Hawkins, 1979:665)

Table 4. Predictability of Genitive Type from Parameters of Verb Phrase and Adposition

SVO & Pr ---	NG	96%
SOV & Po ---	GN	88%
VSO & Pr ---	NG	96%

(my own count from Greenberg 1965)

languages in Hawkins' study. Moreover, both GN languages are also AN languages, suggesting that GN word order in the noun phrase implies AN word order, but not the converse.

Thus, AN word order is not nearly so exceptional in SVO languages as it may first seem. As for prehead genitives, the opposite seems to be true, especially if one combines main clause word order with adposition as a predictor of noun phrase word order as is done in Table 4. This formulation allows predictions to be made for SVO languages that are as strong as those for the more harmonic SOV and VSO languages. Clearly, since English is an SVO language with prepositions, the prehead genitives that exist in English are marked as only 4% of attested languages of its type also have these.

Core Grammar

Since our typological analysis above has shown prehead genitives to be marked in an SVO langauge like English, we would expect to find principles of universal grammar that would also characterize this structure as marked. Initially, if we examine the English VP and NP, in which complements normally follow the head verb or head noun, English must be described as a primarily right-branching language as many, such as Chomsky (1986), maintain. Therefore, prehead genitives, as they are left-branching adjuncts, can be considered marked. Such a characterization concurs with the typological analysis. However, the additional terminology used to describe adjuncts in X-bar configurations, namely "specifier," allows for adjuncts to occur on either side of the head. Though Lightfoot (1979) has suggested the metagrammatical relevancy of such terminology in positing that the presence of a particular grammatical category on the specifier side of the head implies the presence of another category on the complement side, Hawkins (1982) has shown that no such relationship exists; the presence of one category such as DET (determiner) on the specifier side of the head implies nothing about what categories are to be found on the complement side.

Jackendoff (1977) too has noticed the limitations of this terminology:

> This terminology is suitable for discussion of English, though not perhaps for other languages, since it calls the direct object in an SOV langauge part of a specifier, not of complement. ... It must be understood, therefore, that *the distinction between specifier and complement is to regarded here as of no theoretical significance, but only a convenience*. (1977:37 emphasis mine)

The concepts of specifier and complement, therefore, seem to add nothing to the notion of markedness within the English NP since the terms themselves are not metagrammatical, but are instead, devices necessitated in the description of English or a language like it.[2]

The Study

Accepting that prehead NN modification is marked typologically, implicationally, and possibly in terms of generative grammar, one of the questions that presents itself is whether nonnative speakers, assumed to be engaging linguistic universals as they learn the language, will produce these marked constructions with the same frequency that native speakers do. Of course, the bigger question concerns what it is about English that requires or at least allows the use of such marked constructions in place of their unmarked, N prep N counterparts in the first place. Although this study makes no direct attempt to investigate the second question, it does, based upon the results of the following study, offer an answer for the first question.

The hypothesis investigated was this:

> When confronted with the opportunity to construct a GN construction or its N prep N counterpart, nonnative speakers will show a greater preference for the unmarked prepositional construction than will native speakers.

Materials and Procedures

As mentioned before, the constructions under consideration were ten, even-stressed, noun-noun constructions without "s" and their prepositional paraphrases. All were found in the campus newspaper of the University of Kansas in Lawrence in the prehead genitive form. In order to ensure that the noun phrases were interpretable in the limited context of the sentence and to make sure that the original vocabulary and syntax would not prove too complex for nonnative speakers, slight changes were made in the vocabulary and syntax of the sentence in which the constructions were found. These revised sentences were then placed on a two page questionnaire along with four distractors. The noun phrases were disassembled and placed below the sentence on the questionnaire for the test subjects to reconstruct. (See appendix.)

The questionnaires were administered over a period of two weeks to 60 native speakers and 24 nonnative speakers who were students at the University of Kansas. An ANOVA analysis was then done.

Results

Table 5 shows the overall mean preferences for the unmarked NP by both native and nonnative speakers. Although both groups constructed the marked, prehead genitive a majority of the time, the nonnatives were significantly more likely than the native speakers to construct the unmarked, prepositional construction. The native and nonnative means are .36 and .48 respectively.

Table 5. Mean Preferences for the Unmarked Prepositional Construction, Native versus Nonnative Subjects

	native	nonnative
X =	.36	.48
n =	60	24
		(F=16.58, p < .001)
SD =	.36	.26

Table 6. Native and Nonnative Preferences for the Unmarked Prepositional Construction by Adjunct Type

	native	nonnative
Group 1 (locative)		
NP'S	native	nonnative
1. kitchen windows/windows in the kitchen	.37	.71
2. team membership/membership on the team	.63	.33
10. campus speaker/speaker on campus	.33	.71
Average:	.44	.58
Group 2 (descriptive)		
NP'S	native	nonnative
4. KU freshman/freshman from KU	.03	.25
5. campus community/community of the campus	.03	.50
6. door passes/passes for the door	.10	.25
7. White House spokesman/spokesman for the White House	.22	.33
9. military equipment/equipment for the military	0	.13
Average:	.08	.30
Group 3 (discourse dependent)		
NP'S	native	nonnative
3. speech security/security at the speech	.98	.75
8. press attention/attention from the press	.87	.88
Average:	.93	.82

Table 6 lists all ten noun phrases divided into three groups. Group one, the least cohesive of the three groups, is composed of genitives containing locative adjuncts.[3] The native speakers showed some tendency (X=.44) to reconstruct the unmarked noun phrase. Group two is composed of genitives with descriptive adjuncts. For this group, native speakers showed almost no inclination to reconstruct the noun phrase in the unmarked manner (X=.08). The nonnatives roughly mirror this pattern. Group three is composed of two noun phrases referred to here as discourse dependent. Both

Table 7. Preferences for the Unmarked Prepositional Construction and Native Language Genitive Type

		native	non. GN	non. NG
Sentences 1-10	X =	.36	.51	.47
	n =	60	9	15
		(F=8.59, p< .001)		

natives and nonnatives overwhelmingly preferred the unmarked permutation with these noun phrases.

Finally, Table 7 concerns the genitive type of the nonnative speakers' languages and whether this effected their preference for noun phrase type in English. The results show there to be a significant effect. Inexplicably, native language genitive type was significantly related to choosing the opposite type in English. In other words, a nonnative speaker with GN word order in his own language had a significantly greater tendency to choose N prep N genitive word order in English than did the subject whose native language type paralleled the unmarked, N prep N form of English.

Discussion

First of all, these noun phrases all appeared in the marked, prehead adjunct form in the newspaper from which they were taken. The fact that they were reformulated in the unmarked prepositional form to any degree suggests that whatever it is that accounts for the presence of these marked constructions in English is to be found in the extra-grammatical, communicative aspects of language, aspects which were obviously lacking in the context of the study. Secondly, whatever these aspects are which override principles of grammatical markedness, the native speakers of this study seemed to be more aware of them than the nonnative speakers were, for the former were less likely to reformulate the noun phrases in the unmarked manner. Additionally, the fact that the native speaker subjects showed a greater standard deviation for the individual test items (SD=.36) than the nonnative speakers did (SD=.26) suggests that the nonnative speakers were not as sensitive to the fact that the extra-grammatical influences vary with the particular noun phrase.

Before discussing extra-grammatical influences, grammatical ones will be discussed. In comparing groups one and two, it can be seen that the subjects were more likely to place locative adjuncts in a prepositional phrase after the head than they were to place descriptive ones there. It may well be that since adverbials of place normally follow the direct object or the object of a preposition in the verb phrase, this same pattern seems analogically proper in the noun phrases. This may be especially true if the noun phrase is post verbal as it was in all three sentences containing the noun phrases of group one. In fact, for the nonnative speakers, there may even be some structural ambiguity in some cases. A construction such as #1, "windows in the kitchen", though clearly a single, complex noun phrase for the native speakers in the context of sentence 1 (see appendix), might well have been seen by many nonnative subjects as a noun phrase followed by an adverbial of place, just as it clearly is in a sentence such as, "Please put the windows in the kitchen." This sort of interpretation would account for the rather high mean score for the nonnative subjects on this item (X=.71).

In accounting for the native subjects' placing almost no descriptive adjuncts after the head in group 2 (Average X=.08), the influence of adjective-noun constructions is obvious: the descriptive adjuncts in this study function like overtly marked adjectives and thus seem appropriate to precede the head. But in addition, the extra-grammatical influence of speech community or idiom seems to be at work. That the nonnative speakers were much more likely to place adjuncts, especially descriptive ones, in posthead prepositional phrases than natives were, shows them to be less familiar with the marked constructions sanctioned by the speech community. Such grammatically marked constructions as #10, "campus speaker", #4, "KU freshman", and #5, "campus community", are all part of university idiom. I maintain that it is a lack of familiarity with these terms and their functions which helps to account for the greater tendency of nonnatives to place these adjuncts after the head. In other words, less sensitive to extra-grammatical influences of idiom and speech community than native speakers are, nonnative speakers must base their reconstructions more exclusively upon grammatical principles. Since the markedness under investigation in these noun phrases is uniquely relevant to the grammatical domain, it is no wonder that reconstructions conforming to those of the nonnative speakers are more reflective of grammatical universal constraints than those of the natives.

Though the original discourse context was reduced to a single sentence on the questionnaire and this lack of context probably influenced the way the subjects responded to all of the noun phrases, the effect of this missing context is most dramatically seen in group three. The two noun phrases in this group, one containing a locative adjunct and the other a descriptive one, may well have seemed opaque as noun-noun constructions in the limited context of a sentence. Perhaps this is why both native and nonnative speakers overwhelmingly constructed the unmarked prepositional constructions in these two noun phrases. They may have felt that the prepositions present in the unmarked, posthead constructions contained information necessary for interpretation of the noun phrase.

Conclusion

The point of discussing the speech community and the context of discourse is to emphasize that marked, prehead noun modifiers in English owe a great part of their ubiquity to the domains of idiom and discourse, areas outside of the sentence domain of universal grammar or language typology. Such an extra-grammatical source for marked noun-noun constructions would be consistent with the proposals of Li (1975) and Downing (1977) who maintain that the constructions are a form of "telegraphic speech" formed "on the basis of relationships which the speaker perceives to be significant for his classification" (Downing 1977). Thus, the "significance" of the "relationship" between the elements "campus" and "speaker" in the marked construction 'campus speaker" in group one may be due to the context of the university speech community. Once one is a part of this speech community and hence familiar with the social and cultural context, such marked, telegraphic speech is licensed. One consistently recognizes the significant relationship between the two elements of the collocation.

For nonnative speakers, however, such an awareness of significant relationships is likely to be lacking. Nonnative speakers, often new to the American campus and culture and linguistically limited, are for a time only marginal members of the speech community. The contextually significant relationship that allows for such a grammatically marked collocation escapes them, so they construct a noun phrase according to grammatical principles, principles which yield unmarked forms. If this is the case, that speakers ignorant of the speech community idiom will produce unmarked forms, then one would expect native speakers who are unfamiliar with this idiom to likewise produce the unmarked noun phrases. It would be interesting to look at the reconstruction of these same noun phrases by native speakers who have had little or no exposure to the university speech community.

In contrast to the noun phrases of groups one and two discussed above, the significant relationship that obtains between the head and adjunct of the two noun phrases in group three is not determined by the broad context of the speech community. "Speech security", for example, though found in the newspaper in this marked form, was reconstructed in this way by both native speakers and nonnative speakers to only a very limited degree. It appears that the significant relationship that was established in the original context of the newspaper in which the noun phrase was found was not reestablished in the questionnaire. The single sentence was not a sufficient discourse context. Since both groups appear to be sensitive to the absence of the discourse context that licenses the marked construction, one wonders whether both groups would be as sensitive to its presence. A study similar to this one, but providing a discourse context approximating the original newspaper article in which the respondents could reconstruct the noun phrases, would be a step toward discovering how context of discourse can establish the significant relationship that sanctions marked NN constructions and whether or not this relationship is recognized by nonnative speakers.

Finally, as in the results of the Mazurkewich study discussed earlier in which it was maintained that previous exposure to grammatically marked forms and an awareness of stylistical markedness were at play, this study too indicates that results are never free from extra-grammatical influences. No matter how objective and grammatically focused tests are designed to be, subjects must provide comprehensive, linguistic responses, responses generated not only by the grammatical principles to which UG or typological universals apply, but by principles derived from the social context and the context of the discourse. Thus, though a particular approach to the study of language characterizes a certain permutation of a phrase as marked, this markedness only holds within a certain domain of the language, in this case, the grammar. If characterization of preposition stranding and NN genitives as grammatically marked is correct, then their acceptability and even prevalence in language use must be due to other linguistic domains. These domains, namely idiom and context, render grammatically marked constructions the status of fluent and correct English.

Notes

1. Vennemann (1973), for example, feels that fronted stress in indicative of a noun-noun construction having compound status in that the construction has undergone the same sort of historical stress shift that characterizes lexical English nouns. Jespersen (1940:VI:140) has a similar point of view. However, there seem to be many exceptions. "Night plunge", for example, a front-stressed collocation occurring in the university newspaper from which all the noun phrases in this study were taken, appears to this native speaker as a nonce formation seldom, if ever, encountered by the average native speaker. Furthermore, it is difficult to interpret out of context. Does it mean 'plunge at night' or 'plunge into the night'? Compare the interpretability of this front-stressed construction to the even stressed 'ocean plunge'. The latter seems much more easily interpretable.

   Marchand (1969) maintains that the permanency of the lexical relation obtaining between head and adjunct is what determines stress and hence compound status, but can one argue that the front-stressed "mountain lion" involves a more permanent lexical relation between head and adjunct than the evenly stressed construction "mountain ash"? Both constructions do not merely describe a referent, but actually name it.

   Consequently, how can one consider such front-stressed constructions as "night plunge" and "mountain lion" to have compound status or semi-lexical status as distinct from the purely syntactic status of even-stressed "mountain ash" or "evening stroll"? Although the distinction between compounds and genitives may be a worthwhile distinction to make, it must certainly involve more criteria than simply stress pattern.

2. Another problem in reconciling typologically based markedness characterizations with those of generative grammar concerns the differing terminology and the labeling of particular grammatical constructions that result. Typological universals are usually described using the traditional parts of speech wherein prehead adjuncts such as those discussed above are designated as adjectives or nouns according to their morphology. Generative grammar, on the other hand, distinguishes between these adjuncts in terms of X-bar conventions (Chomsky, 1970; Jackendoff, 1977), and a particular adjunct is distinguished from others through its ability to specify a particular head, i.e., N''', N'', N'. Therefore, what has been described as an adjectival construction or a genitive construction in this paper so far does not correspond to what is designated by these terms in the theory of generative grammar. In Chomsky (1970) and Jackendoff (1977) genitive constructions are described as those composed of an N''' specifier of an N''' head. Typically these are the morphologically overt constructions with "s", as in "Fred's house". Other NN constructions which do not include "s" are not referred to as genitives at all, and instead the unmarked noun functions as adjunct appear under and adjectival node A or AP in spite of its morphology. To use terminology in Jackendoff (1977:58), I think he would label constructions containing adjuncts that function adjectivally as "restrictive modifiers", while adjuncts that are "tightly bound to the head" would be "functional arguments". The former are constructions such as 'stone wall' or 'English teacher' (teacher from England), while the latter are constructions such as 'law office' or 'English teacher' (teacher of English), both of which carry fronted stress.

   In this scheme of things, all prehead modifiers have corresponding posthead modifiers: genitives with "s" with nonrestrictive clauses, NN collocations containing restrictive modifiers with N prep N constructions containing restrictive modifiers, and NN collocations containing functional arguments with N prep N constructions containing functional arguments. In Jackendoff's X-bar framework, genitives and nonrestrictive modifiers are adjuncts of N''', restrictive modifiers adjuncts of N'', and functional arguments are adjuncts of N'. However, the relationship from one side of the head to the other is hardly one to one. Though "Fred's house", a nonrestrictive modifier, may well map onto "the house, which is Fred's", a construction such as "girls' school" seems unlikely to map onto "school, which is for girls". A more likely paraphrase is "school for girls", a construction containing a prepositional restrictive modifier of an N''. But even this is not clear cut. "Girls' school" itself may be neither a nonrestrictive or restrictive modifier in an X-bar framework. Given the fronted stress of this construction, "girls'" may well be an adjunct of an N' and therefore a functional argument. Thus, X-bar conventions may label the same adjunct a functional argument on one side of the head and a restrictive modifier on the other. Similar incongruities arise with bare adjunct constructions such as 'stone wall' and 'law office' and their prepositional counterparts. As for the term 'genitive', X-bar terminology restricts it to constructions containing proper nouns of animate reference with "s". Other "s" collocations such as "tomorrow's forecast" would be said to contain a restrictive modifier and therefore would not be genitives.

3. It can be argued that separation of these adjuncts into locative and descriptive is problematic. Locative adjunct number 2, for example, "(on the) team" in "team membership/membership on the team" is locative perhaps only in a figurative sense. Certainly it is not in a literal sense. Moreover, this construction does not really pattern with any of the three groups very well. The native speakers treated it almost as a discourse dependent construction as in group 3 while the nonnative speakers treated it as they did descriptive adjuncts in group 2.

However, it must be borne in mind that I did not choose these particular constructions for the study because of their locative or descriptive meanings; in fact, I did not even recognize them as such at the time. The idea of separating locative from descriptive adjuncts came to me in light of the way the results of the study fell out.

References

Bresnan, J. 1978. "A Realistic Transformational Grammar". *Linguistic Theory and Psychological Reality* ed. by M. Halle, J. Bresnan, and G. Miller, 1-59. Cambridge, MA: MIT Press.

Brown, R., C. Cazden, and U. Bellugi-Klima. 1968. "The Child's Grammar from I to II". *Minnesota Symposium on Child Psychology. vol. 2* ed. by J. Hill, 28-73. Minneapolis: University of Minnesota Press.

Chomsky, N. 1965. *Aspects of the Theory of Syntax. Cambridge, MA: MIT Press.*

Chomsky, N. 1970. "Remarks on Nominalization". *Readings in English Transformational Grammar* ed. by R. Jacobs and P.S. Rosenbaum, 184-221. Waltham, MA: Ginn & Co.

Chomsky, N. 1981. *Lectures on Government and Binding. Dordrecht: Foris.*

Chomsky, N. 1986. Knowledge of Language: Its Nature, Origin, and Use. New York: Praeger.

Clark, H. 1973. "Space, Time, Semantics, and the Child". *Cognitive Development and Acquisition in Language* ed. by T. Moore, New York: Academic Press.

Comrie, B. 1981. *Language Universals and Linguistic Typology*. Chicago: University of Chicago Press.
Downing, P. 1977. "On the Creation and Use of English Compound Nouns". *Language* 53.810-852.
Dulay, H. and M. Burt. 1974. "Natural Sequence in Child L2 Acquisition". *Language Learning* 24.37-53.
Greenberg, J. 1966. *Language Universals with Special Reference to Feature Hierarchies*. The Hague: Mouton.
Hawkins, J. 1979, "Implicational Universals as Predictors of Word Order Change". *Language* 55.618-648.
Hawkins, J. 1982. "Cross-category Harmony, X-bar, and the Predictions of Markedness". *Journal of Linguistics* 18.1-35.
Jackendoff, R. 1977. *X-bar Syntax: A Study of Phrase-Structure*. Cambridge, MA: MIT Press.
Jespersen, O. 1942. *A Modern English Grammar on Historical Principles. Vol. 6*. Copenhagen: Ejnar Munksgaard.
Keenan, E. and B. Comrie. 1977. "Noun Phrase Accessibility and Universal Grammar. *Linguistic Inquiry*. 8.63-99.
Kellerman, E. 1979. "The Problem with Difficulty". *Interlanguage Studies Bulletin* 4.27-48.
Klima, E. and U. Bellugi. 1966. "Syntactic Regularities in the Speech of Children". *Psycholinguistic Papers* ed. by J. Lyons and R. Wales. Edinburgh: University of Edinburgh Press.
Li, C. 1975. *Word Order and Word Order Change*. Austin: University of Texas Press.
Lightfoot, D. 1979. *Principles of Diachronic Linguistics*. Cambridge: Cambridge University Press.
Marchand, H. 1969. *The Categories and Types of Present-day English Word Formation*. Munchen.
Mazurkewich, I. 1984. "The Acquisition of the Dative Alternation by Second Language Learners and Linguistic Theory". *Language Learning* 34.91-109.
Mazurkewich, I. 1985. "Syntactic Markedness and Language Acquisition". *Studies in Second Language Acquisition* 7.15-36.
Rutherford, W., ed. 1984. *Language Universals and Second Language Acquisition*. Amsterdam: John Benjamins.
Van Reimsdijk, H. and E. Williams. 1986. *Introduction to the Theory of Grammar*. Cambridge, MA: MIT Press.
Vennemann, T. 1974. "Topics, Subjects, and Word Order: from SXV to SVX via TVX". *Historical Linguistics* ed. by J. Anderson and C. Jones. Amsterdam: North Holland.
White, L. 1982. *Grammatical Theory and Language Acquisition*. Dordrecht: Foris.
White, L. 1987. "Markedness and Second Language Acquisition: The Question of Transfer". *Studies in Second Language Acquisition* 9.261-268.
Zobl, H. 1983. "Markedness and the Projection Problem". *Language Learning* 33.293-313.

Appendix

The Ten Test Sentences as They Appeared on the Questionnaire
(minus the four distractors)

1. She said that the explosion broke all of the ______ -windows- -kitchen- (the, in)
2. Last night, two senators introduced a petition that would end Smith's ______. -team- -membership- (the, on)
3. Because the Senate feared violent protest, they provided another $800 for ______. -security- -speech- (the, at)
4. Two ______ -KU- -freshmen- (from) took an unexpected swim last night when the car they were in rolled into Clinton Lake.
5. Mr. Smith thinks that the ______ -community- -campus- (the, of) should know about this man's reputation.
6. Members of the public may attend the speech if they have ______. -passes- -door- (the, for)
7. A ______ -spokesman- -White House- (the, for) said that the administration was considering diplomatic steps in response to yesterday's shooting in East Germany.
8. Mary Jones said that she couldn't remember any other speaker who had drawn so much ______. -press- -attention- (the, from)
9. The U.S. observer was photographing ______ -equipment- -military- (the, of) when he was shot.
10. John Young was the only ______ -campus- -speaker- (on) who drew such a large audience.

The Null-Prep Phenomenon:

The Interaction of Linguistic Theory and Second Language Acquisition Data

Elaine C. Klein
Queens College

In the acquisition process, adult second language (L2) learners of English often omit the preposition from a WH question or relative clause requiring either a pied-piping or preposition stranding construction. Learners therefore produce such sentences as those in (1),

(1) a. **Which* movie were the girls talking yesterday?
b. *Here's the movie (*which/that/Ø*) the girls were talking yesterday.

instead of the required forms as in (2) and (3):

(2) PIED-PIPING:
a. *About which* movie were the girls talking yesterday?
b. Here's the movie *about which* the girls were talking yesterday.

(3) PREPOSITION-STRANDING:
a. Which movie were the girls talking *about* yesterday?
b. Here's the movie (*which/that/Ø*) the girls were talking *about* yesterday.

I am calling the omission of the preposition in constructions such as (1), the "null-prep phenomenon". In this paper, I will show: 1) how discovery of this null-prep phenomenon in the L2 grammar motivated inquiry into a neglected area of linguistic research, and 2) how the findings from this linguistic research have created new questions for UG markedness-based accounts of second language acquisition (SLA).

L2 studies of pied-piping and preposition stranding have attempted to test a markedness hypothesis by determining whether the markedness values for piping and stranding correlate with acquisition order. According to linguists such as Van Reimsdijk (1978) and Hornstein and Weinberg (1981), preposition stranding is a comparatively marked form. Pied-piping, in turn, is its unmarked counterpart.

The near-universal agreement (but see, for example, Stowell 1981) on these particular markedness values has led SLA researchers to utilize pied-piping and preposition stranding (hereafter, piping and stranding) to test the relationship between L2 acquisition and UG markedness. One such UG claim involves a strong Developmental Hypothesis where an L2 learner is argued to begin acquisition by setting her parameters at the unmarked values or initial state, S_o, as does a child learning the L1. Thus, under this hypothesis, learners would be expected to exhibit piping, the unmarked form, before stranding. Alternatively, the Contrastive Hypothesis proposes that UG effects interact with L1 markedness settings; that is, the L2 learner initially sets her parameters at the L1 values and resets to the L2 on the basis of positive evidence from the target language input. Here, L2 learners' acquisition of piping and stranding would vary, depending on the relationship between the particular L1 and L2 markedness settings involved.

To investigate these hypotheses, several L2 researchers have tested whether pied-piping appears before preposition stranding in the acquisition process and if there are variable results according to a subject's L1. Some relevant studies include Mazurkewich (1984) and Bardovi-Harlig (1987) who come to different conclusions, for reasons which will not be elaborated here (but see Klein 1990, for details). However, these researchers similarly show that before either piping or stranding appears, many adult L2 learners of English omit the relevant preposition in these constructions. The omission of the preposition in these studies, however, is explained away as practice test biases[1] or, more likely, subcategorization errors. Concerning the latter, Bardovi-Harlig suggests that subjects leaving out the preposition in questions and relatives have not yet learned that a particular verb requires a prepositional argument.

To further investigate whether this phenomenon could be solely attributed to subcategorization errors or practice test influences, I pilot-tested fifty-three adult L2 learners of English at Hunter College of the City University of New York. Subjects from a variety of L1 backgrounds were divided into two broad proficiency levels, mid-beginners and mid-intermediates. In a grammaticality judgement and correction task, subjects were first given practice test sentences which included some verbs that required prepositions and others that did not. Then they were asked to judge declarative sentences, and corresponding questions and relative clauses. Verbs requiring *prepositions were tested and these prepositions were omitted in all targeted sentences*. Thus, subjects were presented with sentences as shown in (4):[2]

(4) a. The delivery boy applied a new job last week.
b. Which job did the delivery boy apply last week?
c. This is the job (which/that/Ø) the delivery boy applied last week.

If a subject judged the declarative (4a) as correct, it was presumed that the subject did not know the correct subcategorization features for that verb; therefore, the related question (4b) and relative clause (4c) were not examined for that particular subject. However, if a subject judged the declarative as incorrect, and corrected it by adding the required preposition, then the related question and relative were examined. If the same subject accepted (4b) and/or (4c) as correct (i.e. without the required preposition), then these were counted as null-prep data. The results are shown in Table 1.

Table 1. Acceptance of Null-Prep in questions and relative clauses

	Questions	Relative Clauses	Total Average
(mid) beginners	69.0%	76.0%	72.5%
(mid) intermed.	36.0%	57.5%	46.8%

At the beginning level, subjects who showed correct subcategorization in particular declaratives accepted null-prep at a rate of 69% in the corresponding questions and 76% in the corresponding relatives. The intermediate-level subjects accepted null-prep at a rate of 36% in questions and 57.5% in relatives, showing a clear developmental pattern.

Importantly, there were no apparent differences among various L1 backgrounds, some of which were postpositional and some prepositional. Also included were languages with only pied-piping (i.e. not stranding), suggesting that transfer of what has been called the unmarked form is not a significant factor in the results.[3]

These results clearly indicate that null-prep is not a subcategorization error, but that it represents an early stage in the acquisition of piping or stranding. Further, since the results show consistent responses across different L1s, the Contrastive Hypothesis is not supported here. And finally, the Developmental Hypothesis can only be supported if it can be shown that null-prep is even less marked than pied-piping.

A linguistic investigation of null-prep now becomes essential if we are to determine the extent to which these findings in the L2 grammar correlate with predictions of UG markedness settings, if they do at all. That is, can we show that null-prep is a relatively unmarked form? It has to be shown first, however, that null-prep is a true linguistic construction since, it has been generally claimed that for both L1 and L2 acquisition, each stage of a learner's linguistic development represents a structure possible in natural languages (for example, see Adjemian 1976; Liceras 1985; White 1987).

Although rarely attested and even more sparsely examined in the linguistic literature, it appears to be the case that null-prep occurs in, at least, one of the world's languages. According to Comrie (personal communication), colloquial Brazilian Portuguese requires a full prepositional phrase in a simple declarative sentence, but allows omission of the preposition in the corresponding relative clause as in (5):[4]

(5) *Colloquial Brazilian Portuguese* (from Thomas 1969:302):

a. *Falam da moça.*
They-talk about-the girl.
'They talk about the girl.'

b. *Aquella é a moça que falam tanto...*
That is the girl that they-talk so much...
'That's the girl that they talk so much about...'

It is clear, then, that L2 learners are creating a structure that is within the realm of natural language phenomena. It becomes important, now, to further examine null-prep typologically and syntactically to see how linguistic theory can shed light on the acquisition phenomenon. A preliminary typological investigation was therefore conducted to see how the construction might fit into a markedness framework, as determined by some of the broad markedness criteria summarized in Moravcsik and Wirth (1987), particularly cross-linguistic frequency and syntactic "complexity".[5]

Examining the phenomenon cross-linguistically, I have found that null-prep occurs in languages other than colloquial Brazilian Portuguese. It is exhibited, under various conditions, in the following prepositional languages, among others: colloquial Puerto Rican Spanish, Catalan, Modern Greek, Modern Hebrew, Quebecois, Modern French and in standard Chinese, 17th c. French, Old English, and Roviana, a language spoken in New Georgia, Solomon Islands. In these languages, except for some rare idiosyncratic exceptions, null-prep is restricted to relative clauses. Examples of null-prep in Puerto Rican Spanish and Greek appear in (6) and (7):

(6) *Colloquial Puerto Rican Spanish*

a. *Ella vive en esa casa.*
She lived in that house.

b. *Esta es la casa que ella vivo.*
That is the house that she lived.
'That's the house that she lived in.'

(7) *Colloquial Modern Greek* (from Maling, 1977)

a. *Aphesa to vilió páno stó trapézi.*
I-left the book on the table.

b. *Aphtó eine to trapezi pou áphesa to vivlio.*
This is the table that I-left the book.
'This is the table that I left the book on.'

Typologically, the trend seems to show that null-prep is fairly frequent within a sub-set of prepositional or comp-initial languages — those which have clitics and weak prepositions and which also exercise a resumptive pronoun strategy[6] in the relevant PP, as in the ungrammatical English equivalent, "The man that I am talking to him".

Interestingly, in some postpositional or comp-final languages, a phenomenon similar to null-prep is exhibited. In both Japanese and Korean, for example, there is obligatory omission of the postposition in relative clauses. At the same time, this postposition is mandatory in declaratives and questions, exactly parallel to the null-prep construction in prepositional languages. The following example is from Japanese:[7]

(8) a. *Watashi-wa sono ie ni sunde iru.*
I -top that house in-loc live T-present
'I live in that house.'

b. *Sore-ga* *watashi-ga* *sunde-iru* *ie.*
That-nom I-nom live-pres house.
'That's the house I live in.'

Omission of the adposition, then, occurs across both comp-initial and comp-final language groups. More extensive research may show this to be a related phenomenon.

When we examine null-prep typologically, there appear to be correlations between null-prep and the following characteristics in the languages where it occurs: Null-prep occurs only in relative clauses, never in questions; null-prep relatives are always introduced by an invariant complementizer, never a relative pronoun; null-prep always alternates with a resumptive pronoun; null-prep only occurs in languages with clitics or clitic-like prepositions; null-prep only occurs in languages which permit null object pronouns (*pro*, as described by Rizzi 1986).

The next investigation involved a close syntactic examination of the structure in two divergent languages: Brazilian Portuguese and Greek (see Klein 1990). On the basis of my findings, the following analysis is proposed: Null-prep is argued to be a base-generated empty category in non-movement relative clauses. It occurs when a weak preposition (see footnote 11) licenses its null object (*pro*) and then becomes null itself by cliticizing to it. This results from the interaction of three related parameters.

Specifically rejecting a narrow piping/stranding parameter with a binary switch between two values, I posit three broad interacting parameters which result in all possible relative clause options across prepositional (for now) languages: pied-piping, preposition stranding (in WH-movement languages) and resumptive pronouns, null-prep, and "intransitive stranding" [8] (in non-WH-movement languages).[9] The three parameters, with their related markedness values, are shown in Table 2.

Table 2. The parameters for relative clauses in prepositional languages

Parameter I.	+/− WH-movement[10]
Parameter II.	+/− licensing/proper government of an empty object by a preposition, where + = M; − = U
Parameter III.	+/− weak preposition[11] where + = U; − = M

Notes: M = the marked value; U = the unmarked value.

To summarize, it is argued that the markedness settings of relative clause constructions are determined by the interaction of these three parameters. Thus, in WH-movement constructions, pied-piping is unmarked, since the construction results from the U values of parameters II and III, above. Preposition stranding is more marked since it involves a strong preposition, the M setting of parameter III.

Crucial to the discussion here, the resumptive pronoun is the least marked setting of the non-movement options in II and III (i.e. The weak clitic-preposition can only license a *lexical* object; thus the parametric setting for II is U. In addition, the clitic-preposition (=weak) reflects the U setting of parameter III.). Null-prep is more marked than the resumptive option since it results from the M setting of parameter II (i.e. the preposition licenses its empty object). Intransitive stranding is the most marked of all, resulting from the M values of both II and III. Thus, for non-movement relatives, the markedness order is as follows:

Resumptive pronouns (UU) -->
Null-prep (MU) -->
Intransitive stranding (MM)

It is important to note that null-prep cannot be analyzed as a core construction in movement languages since proper government of a trace by a weak preposition or clitic is not possible (see footnote 11). This explains why null-prep is not found in questions involving WH-movement. In such constructions, null-prep would represent an illegal (or very highly marked) option and would only occur as a peripherial construction.

This occurs in English in sentences like those in (9) and (10).

(9) a. She graduated in 1988.
*She graduated 1988.
b. (In) which year did she graduate?
c. … the year (that) she graduated

(10) a. He left for that reason.
*He left that reason.
b. *(For) which reason did he leave?
c. … the reason (that) she left

These "bare NP" constructions (see Larson 1985), although superficially like null-prep, are different from the latter in many ways (see Klein 1990). They can occur in movement constructions with strong prepositions, are lexically-determined, and are argued to be idiosyncratic structures in the periphery.

It is now time to examine how this linguistic study, originally motivated by L2 data, can help further our understanding of the relevant SLA questions. That is, we can now utilize the linguistic analysis of null-prep to formulate possible explanations for the null-prep phenomenon in the L2 grammar of English.

Three possible explanations are offered, among others:

(a) L2 learners may be guided by UG and assume non-movement for piping or stranding constructions. In the absence of positive evidence for the least marked option (i.e. resumptive pronouns) in English, learners choose null-prep, the next option in the markedness hierarchy of non-movement relatives. The existence of null-prep in L2 questions is a problem for this explanation since, as we recall, null-prep has not been thus far attested in the questions of natural languages. UG may be saved if it can be said that L2 learners are treating questions as non-movement constructions (which are, at least, potentially possible in natural languages); however, this hypothesis will continue to be a problem for UG unless it can be shown that L1 learners begin the acquisition of questions with non-movement (i.e. that non-movement is the unmarked setting of the relevant parameter).[12]

(b) L2 learners may be misanalyzing the input of English. That is, they misconstrue "bare NPs" and utilize a peripheral construction to set core parameters for the null-prep construction. If these learners are creating a possible grammar (i.e. obeying UG), they are setting parameters to create the wrong possible grammar relative to the language they are exposed to. Thus, they are doing something different from what L1 children do, suggesting that part of UG is missing.

(c) L2 learners are utilizing adult problem-solving or processing mechanisms rather than parameter setting. Under this explanation, they are learning the language piecemeal, depending on local options. Adult strategies instigate learners to assume that the absence of a preposition in clause-initial position (in cases of stranding), or in clause-final position (in cases of piping), is evidence that prepositions are optional in English. What appear to be omitted prepositions may also be construed as further evidence of "bare NPs" throughout the grammar, a case of overgeneralization. This is in contrast to children learning L1 English where UG provides them with knowledge of the dependency relationship between stranding and piping (as a single fact about the language), and with a mechanism to acquire the core as distinct from the periphery.

Further research is clearly needed to sort out these explanations. Specifically, tests of L2 learners can determine the existence of movement/non-movement in both relatives and questions (e.g. tests of subjacency violations, crossover violations, parasitic gaps). It will also be important to test child learners of English as L1 and L2, as well as learners of L1s and L2s other than English — languages which do not have "bare NPs" in the periphery from which learners may be incorrectly overgeneralizing or triggering core parameters, and languages which do not have both piping and stranding to encourage illicit processing or problem-solving strategies. And finally, it will be important to further examine the acquisition of core versus peripheral structures in both the L1 and L2 to further support the hypothesis that somewhat different mechanisms are at work for children in contrast to adults.

Exactly how those mechanisms differ is the critical acquisition question. This research clearly indicates that the UG markedness questions, as they are currently posed in L2 studies, need to be refined and extended. We must now ask to what extent second language learners are guided by UG, if at all. It is probable that "UG or not UG"[13] is not the ultimate question. My research suggests that, at least, part of UG may be missing and it will be up to L2 researchers to continue to explore which part that may be, as well as why and how this happens.

On a broader scale, null-prep in L2 grammars has opened some new areas of inquiry and offers an example of how second language acquisition research can interact with, and help inform, linguistic theory — in particular parameter and markedness theory, as Gair 1988 suggests. It was shown that acquisition research involving traditional markedness criteria requires cross-linguistic and close syntactic analyses of the constructions being investigated. In the particular case of null-prep, this investigation of an acquisition phenomenon has revealed a comparatively ignored natural language structure which needs to be further investigated within linguistic theory.

Notes

1. That is, Mazurkewich argues that her subjects could have modeled their (null-prep) answers after practice test sentences in which verbs without prepositional complements were presented.

2. Related sentences such as these appeared in random order and were interspersed with filler sentences which included prepositions.

3. This pilot study has been replicated with 196 adult non-native speakers of English at the American Language Institute of New York University. Subjects were from 18 L1s, and 40 native speakers served as controls. A 5-point confidence-rating scale was included where subjects had to indicate "how sure" they were of their answers. These results are reported in Klein (1990), and clearly support the findings of my pilot study. The robust null-prep data are further strengthened with the confidence rating scale where subjects indicated that they were "very sure" of their null-prep responses.

4. Comrie (personal communication) suggests that further exploration would probably show that null-prep is exhibited in other (probably colloquial) languages as well.

5. It would appear that null-prep is highly marked on the basis of its infrequency in the world's languages. However, the frequency criteron for markedness will never be conclusive since it is not possible, in principle, to study all the possible languages of the world.

6. Sells (1981) makes a distinction between intrusive and resumptive pronouns, the latter restricted to a construction involving operator-bound variables. I am not making this distinction here, and include both types of pronouns under "resumptives".

7. When this rule similarly operates in Quechua, deletion of the postposition is allowed to leave the sentence ambiguous. Ambiguities are also evident in other examples, with potential implications for violation of the universal principle on Recoverabilty of Deletion (see Chomsky 1964, 1986; Chomsky and Lasnik 1977, among others).

8. This refers to the option where a preposition may remain overt and license its empty object (*pro*) in a non-movement construction (see Vinet 1979; Zribi-Hertz 1984). By contrast, preposition stranding in languages like English and Dutch, for example, is always a WH-movement construction. Bouchard (1984) argues that non-movement stranding only occurs with "strong" prepositions.

9. Resumptives are considered, here, in the general category of non-movement constructions, although there have been arguments presented (see Sells, 1981) for resumptives related to WH-movement.

10. This parameter will be considered "open" (having no markedness values) for the present.

11. "Weak" prepositions are considered, here, as bound morphemes and are very common in the world's languages; for purposes of this analysis, they are being interpreted as clitics and, as such, cannot govern a trace for purposes of satisfying the ECP (i.e. The Empty Category Principle (ECP) requires that a trace be properly governed, where proper government is government by a lexical governor or a local antecedent.) "Strong" prepositions, on the other hand, are not bound to an adjacent word (or empty category) and are very rare; they may be proper governors and, as such, may result in preposition stranding. (See Hornstein and Weinberg 1981 for a different analysis.)

12. This question is currently being investigated by several L1 researchers of English, including Nishigauchi and Roeper (1987), McDaniel and McKee (1989), and Crain (1989).

13. This refers to a paper by du Plessis et al. (1987) titled "UG or not UG, That Is the Question: A Reply to Clahsen and Muysken."

References

Adjemian, C. 1976. "On the Nature of Interlanguage Systems". *Language Learning* 26.297-320.

Bardovi-Harlig K. 1987. "Markedness and Salience in Second Language Acquisition". *Language Learning* 37.385-408.

Bouchard, D. 1984. On the Content of Empty Categories. Dordrecht: Foris.

Bresnan, J. 1971. *The Theory of Complementation in English Syntax*. Doctoral dissertation. Massachusetts Institute of Technology.

Chomsky, N. 1964. *Current Issues in Linguistic Theory*. The Hague: Mouton.

Chomsky, N. 1986. *Knowledge of Language. Its Nature, Origin, and Use*. New York: Praeger.

Chomsky, N. and H. Lasnik. 1977. "Filters and Control". *Linguistic Inquiry* 8.425-504.

Comrie, B. 1981. *Language Universals and Linguistic Typology*. Chicago: U. of Chicago Press.

Crain, S. 1989. "Why Production Precedes Comprehension". Paper presented at the Boston University Conference on Language Development, October, 1989.

du Plessis, J., D. Solin, L. Travis, and L. White. 1987. "UG or not UG, That Is the Question: A Reply to Clahsen and Muysken". *Second Language Research* 3.56-75.

Gair, J. W. 1988. "Kinds of Markedness". *Linguistic Theory in Second Language Acquisition* ed. by S. Flynn and W. O'Neil, 225-250. Dordrecht: Kluwer Academic Publishers.

Hornstein N. and A. Weinberg. 1981. "Case Theory and Preposition Stranding". *Linguistic Inquiry* 12.55-91.

Ingria, R. 1981. *Sentential Complementation in Modern Greek*. Doctoral dissertation, Massachusetts Institute of Technology.

Kayne, R. 1981. "On Certain Differences between French and English". *Linguistic Inquiry* 12.349-371.

Keenan, E.L. and B. Comrie. 1977. "Noun Phrase Accessibility and Universal Grammar". *Linguistic Inquiry* 27.93-108.

Klein, E. 1990. *The Null-prep Phenomenon in Second Language acquisition*. Doctoral dissertation, The Graduate School and University Center, City University of New York.

Larson, R.K. 1985. "Bare-NP Adverbs". *Linguistic Inquiry* 16.595-621.

Liceras, J. 1985. "The Role of Intake in the Determination of Learners' Competence". *Input and Second Language Aquisition* ed. by S. Gass and C. Madden, 354-373. Rowley, MA: Newbury House.

Mazurkewich, I. 1984. "Dative Questions and Markedness". *Universals of Second Language Acquisition* ed. by F. Eckman, L. Bell and D. Nelson, 119-131. Rowley, MA: Newbury House.

Maling, J. 1977. "A Nonrecoverable Deletion". *The Chicago Linguistic Society Book of Squibs Cumulative Index* ed. by S. Fox, W. Beach and S. Philosoph. Chicago Linguistic Society: U. of Chicago.

McDaniel, D. and C. McKee. 1989. "Which Children Did They Show Obey Strong Crossover?" Unpublished ms. U. Mass.

Moravcsik, E. and J. Wirth. 1987. "Markedness - an Overview". *Markedness* ed. by F. Eckman, E. Moravcsik and J. Wirth, 1-12. New York: Plenum Press.

Nishigauchi, T. and T. Roeper. 1987. "Deductive Parameters and the Growth of Empty Categories". *Parameter Setting* ed. by T. Roeper and E. Williams, 91-122. Dordrecht: D. Reidel Publishing Company.

Rizzi, L. 1986. "Null Objects in Italian and the Theory of pro." *Linguistic Inquiry* 17.501-557.

Sells, P. 1981. The Syntax and Semantics of Resumptive Pronouns. Doctoral dissertation, U. Mass.

Stowell, T. 1981. Origins of Phrase Structure. Doctoral dissertation, MIT.

Tarallo, F. 1983. *Relativization strategies in Brazilian Portuguese*. Doctoral dissertation, U. Penn.

Thomas, E.W. 1969. *The Syntax of Brazilian Portuguese*. Nashville: Vanderbilt U. Press.

Van Reimsdijk. H. 1978. *A Case Study in Syntactic Markedness: The Binding Nature of Prepositional Phrases*. Dordrecht: Foris.

Vinet, M-T. 1979. "Dialect Variation and a Restrictive Theory of Grammar: A Study of Intransitive Prepositions in a Variety of French". *Montreal Working Papers in Linguistics. 13.107-125.*

White, L. 1987. "Markedness and Second Language Acquisition: The Question of Transfer". Studies in Second Language Acquisition 9.261-285.

Zribi-Hertz, A. 1984. "Prépositions Orphelines and et Pronoms Nuls". *Recherches Linguistiques* 12.46-91.

Apparent UG Inaccessibility in Second Language Acquisition:

Misapplied Principles or Principled Misapplications?

Gita Martohardjono and James W. Gair
Cornell University

Introduction

In recent years, there has been an increase in the number of studies investigating the role played by principles and parameters of Universal Grammar (UG) in the acquisition of a Second Language (SLA)*. There are currently two diverging positions in the field. On the one hand, there is evidence suggesting that UG principles constrain SLA in ways similar to First Language Acquisition. This position has been advanced by researchers like Ritchie (1978), Liceras (1989), Flynn (1984, 1987, 1988) White (1986, 1989) Bley-Vroman, Felix and Ioup (1988) who might be referred to collectively as the UG-based group. They generally point to effects in SLA that can be related to UG but are not easily attributed to any learning strategy.In addition, some of this research suggests that the effects of the First Language (L1) in SLA are in fact guided by the interplay of differentially set parameters in the learner's L1 and L2. The evidence adduced in these studies thus strongly suggest that UG plays a significant role in SLA.

A second group of researchers testing UG principles focuses on the fact that second language learners rarely attain native speaker proficiency in UG-related phenomena. They generally adduce data showing differences between L1 and L2 learning, for example in areas where certain processing principles are invoked in the L2 but not in the L1 (e.g. Clahsen and Muysken 1988). Alternatively they point to "incompleteness" of acquisition. Bley-Vroman (1989), Schachter (1990) and Johnson (1988). Contrary to the

UG based group, these researchers generally conclude that UG principles are either not accessible, or accessible only in an altered form to adult language learners.

One fact that emerges in several of these studies is that L2 learners perform significantly above chance in recognizing violations of UG principles (cf. Bley-Vroman, Felix and Ioup 1988, Johnson 1988), strongly suggesting that there is in fact a UG effect in SLA. What needs to be explained, then, is why SL learners do not perform as well as native speakers. We propose that this is partly due to the hypothesis space made available by UG itself. Furthermore, we raise the possibility of an "interaction" between the L1 and the L2 which is a more general concept than the notions of "transfer" or "interference" commonly invoked in the literature. We will show that this "interaction" is itself constrained by UG.

The "problem": L1 effects in L2 acquisition

The point on which the two groups of researchers mentioned above diverge seems to be in the interpretation of the role played by the learner's L1 in the acquisition of the L2. For example, Johnson (1988) and Schachter (1988) argue that UG principles which are not instantiated in the L1 (or instantiated in a different way than is required by the L2) become effete in some sense, and are thus inaccessible for the acquisition of an L2 in adulthood. In some sense the L1 is thus viewed as an obstruction to UG-guided acquisition of the L2.

Researchers within the UG-based group also address the question of L1 effects in L2 acquisition. However, their explanation for such effects is itself formulated within a UG-theoretic framework. For example, White (1986) has suggested that the phenomenon known as "transfer" can in some sense be accounted for by the "parameters" aspect of UG theory. Simplifying her position somewhat, we could say that in the absence of evidence, the learner will hypothesize that the L2 is like the L1 as far as any particular parameter settings are concerned. Under this hypothesis it is predicted that in cases where the L1 and the L2 have a particular parameter set differently, "transfer" will result. Flynn (1987) has also proposed that L1 effects in L2 acquisition can best be explained within a UG-based research paradigm. Flynn's position differs from White's in that the learner's initial assumption is not seen to be that of identity between the L1 and the L2. Instead, the L1 is seen as "mediating" in some sense the acquisition of the L2. For example, if for a given parameter there is a mismatch in the settings between the L1 and L2, the learner must reset the parameter. This process thus involves the "reconstruction" of a grammar and may take time.

The General Hypothesis

The account of SLA we propose in this paper accords with that of White and Flynn in several respects: Firstly, we hypothesize that SLA is based on a process of grammar construction rather than the utilization of general learning strategies alone (as suggested for example in Clahsen and Muysken 1986). Secondly, we concur with the idea that the grammars L2 learners construct for the Target Language may initially not be the right one; in particular we will show that certain aspects of the L1 grammar may interact in shaping the learner's grammar (L2). Crucially, however, we suggest that the ways in which L2 grammars diverge from the grammar of the Target Language are themselves constrained by UG. We thus subscribe to the hypothesis that L2 grammars fall within the range of "natural languages" (cf. Selinker 1972; Corder 1967). Our position is not formulated in terms of parameters because so far no parameter-theoretic proposals have been made for the phenomenon we consider. This is not to say, however, that a parametric view is incompatible with ours, and we leave the question open here.

A Methodological Note

An important corollary of our hypothesis concerns methodology: Typically, an SLA experiment will focus on a particular UG principle testing for its effect in the learner's knowledge of the L2 through the learner's judgments of sentences violating the principle. Thus, if the learner shows evidence of knowledge that the ungrammatical sentences are ungrammatical, this is taken to mean that the UG principle tested for is "active". If, on the other hand, the learner does not show knowledge of the ungrammaticality of the sentences, that same principle (and by implication, UG) is taken to be "inactive" or not available to the learner.

While we agree with the general approach of that research, we suggest that in some cases testing UG principles in isolation may be an inadequate measure of the learner's grammatical system. Rather, we propose that the assessment of L2 grammars should involve the simultaneous investigation of several aspects of the learner's competence. Our basic hypothesis is that the failure to observe a UG principle in L2 does not necessarily prove the unavailability of UG or even of that particular principle, but that some crucial prior conditions for its application may not be satisfied in the learner's grammar. The situation we have in mind arises when UG gives several options in the way structures are generated across languages, and when these options instantiate different principles. Suppose, for example, that UG allows structure S to be generated in two ways, A and B, which respectively instantiate principles Pa and Pb. Suppose further that the Target Language requires S to be generated in way A, hence obeys Pa. Learners acquiring this language may have a grammar which generates S in way B, following Pb. In this case, straightforward testing of learners' grammars for observance of Pa may give negative results. However, this does not necessarily mean that the grammar violates Pa, but simply that Pa is not relevant at this point in the acquisition process because the learner does not "recognize" that it applies. The learner's grammar is "incorrect" from the point of view of the Target Grammar, because it has instantiated the wrong option given by UG, but it does not in itself fall outside of what is permitted by UG.

"Movement/no movement" as a test case

One UG phenomenon which may give rise to the situation we have just described is syntactic movement, an aspect of grammar which has been the focus of many SLA studies. What makes movement particularly useful for our purposes is that on the one hand, it is subject to several UG principles, e.g. Subjacency, ECP, but on the other hand, it is in itself optional in terms of its application to specific structures cross-linguistically. For example, as illustrated in table 1. below, the first group of languages uses wh-movement to generate questions, relative clauses, and topics. In the second group, this option is instantiated only for a subset of these structures. Neither Chinese nor Indonesian uses movement to generate wh-questions. Chinese and Indonesian differ from one another in that the former but not the latter uses movement to generate Relative Clauses. Finally, for Topicalization, both

Table 1.

	Wh-questions	Rel. Clauses	Topicalization
English French German	movement	movement	movement
Chinese	no movement	movement	movement/no movement
Indonesian	no movement	no movement	movement/no movement

Chinese and Indonesian (cf. Huang 1980, 1984, Kaswanti Purwo 1981, Martohardjono 1988) may or may not involve movement (i.e. regular vs. "non-gap" topics).

Testing movement principles in L2 grammars

In the SLA studies that test for movement principles, subjects are usually native speakers of an L1 which does not have movement for the particular structure being tested. The underlying assumption is that if UG is available to these learners, thcy should recognize violations of a movement principle regardless of whether movement is used in the L1. We suggest that in this form, the hypothesis is too strong, and that it does not necessarily follow from a UG-based analysis of SLA. In particular, there seems to be an additional learnability issue involved here, namely, that in order to recognize a movement violation in the L2, the learner first needs to identify which structures in the L2 do in fact involve movement. Recall (from table 1) that movement is an option in UG, i.e. nothing in UG forces movement in particular structural configurations.

To recapitulate our specific hypothesis then: since UG leaves unspecified whether certain structures are generated by movement or not (i.e. this is a language- as well as structure-specific option), knowledge regarding the presence or absence of movement in a specific structure in the L2 must be learned/induced. It is thus possible that at some stage during acquisition this knowledge may not yet be available to the L2 learners (or only partially available, e.g. for only a subset of the structures which involve movement in the L2). In other words, it is possible that the L2 grammar does not generate specific structures for the L2 in the particular way required by the L2, while still falling within the boundaries of what is allowed by UG. It is for that reason that judgments of subjacency violations alone are not a reliable measure of the presence or absence of UG in the learner's grammar. Rather, we would expect recognition of Subjacency violations in a particular structure only if the interlanguage grammar at that point generates that structure by movement. What we need, in other words, is a way to assess whether learners' grammars correctly generate certain structures in their L2 by movement. In the next section we outline a set of "movement diagnostics" which may be used for this purpose.

The Diagnostics of Movement

In the theory of Universal Grammar the presence or absence of movement is associated with several corollary phenomena. For example:

a. Movement (but crucially not non-movement) is constrained by Subjacency.
b. Movement gaps are different in nature from non-movement gaps.

More precisely, there are three different types of gaps, *pro*, PRO and "trace", of which only the latter is generated by movement. *pro* occurs in many languages, including Italian, in tensed sentences lacking overt pronouns, such as *pro voglio andare al cinema* 'I want to go to the cinema.' PRO occurs within non-finite domains in so-called "control" sentences, such as *John promised Bill PRO to go to the store*.

Both of these types of empty categories are base-generated. "Traces" or "variables" on the other hand, are generated by syntactic movement in sentences such as questions in English: *What$_i$ did John see t$_i$?*.

All three types of gaps are governed by different principles and modules of UG. However, the structures that we deal with in this paper are non-control finite ones, and thus do not involve PRO. Our concern is only with the difference between "trace" and *pro* as moved and non-moved gaps respectively, in terms of their privileges of occurrence. The particular characteristics of these elements that are of relevance are as follows:

i. "trace" is governed by the ECP ("Empty Category Principle") which requires non-pronominal gaps to be "properly governed", i.e. lexically or by antecedent-government.

ii. *pro* is subject to a different set of principles, namely
   a. licensing conditions (several have been proposed, e.g. "recoverability" by "rich" AGR (cf. Taraldsen 1978; Chomsky 1982); "morphological uniformity" (Jaeggli and Safir 1989)
   b. proper identification (e.g. Generalized Control Rule, (Huang 1984))
   c. Principle B of the Binding Theory: i.e., as a pronoun, it cannot be bound by an antecedent in its governing category (for present purposes, this means its own minimal S)
   d. For languages with Subject-Verb agreement, or no agreement, a universal constraint has been proposed against *pro* in object position (Huang 1984, Raposo 1986).

The theory thus predicts that the use of movement to generate a particular construction crucially carries with it a set of grammatical consequences, both in terms of the specific principles which are relevant to that construction (e.g. Subjacency and ECP), as well as in terms of the nature of the gap that is involved (variable vs. *pro*). In cross-linguistic research it is standard practice to use these consequences as diagnostics to determine whether for a certain construction in a particular language, movement is involved or not. For example, Huang (1984) and Cole (1987) argue that certain structures in Chinese and Imbabura Quecha are not generated by movement because they do not obey Subjacency.

Using movement diagnostics on L2 grammars

Under the hypothesis that L2 grammars are "natural" and hence constrained by UG we can now use the same method to determine whether a given L2 grammar involves movement for a given construction. For example, suppose that there is a point during acquisition at which the L2 grammar does not have movement. We would expect that for that grammar:

i. NP gaps would be filled by *pro* (or possibly PRO since trace can only be created by movement).
ii. Subjacency (a movement principle) is irrelevant (or vacuous)
iii. The ECP is irrelevant (since the only gaps in this grammar are pronominal, and only non-pronominals are subject to the ECP)

iv. Certain object gaps are not allowed, since in this grammar gaps can only be filled by *pro* which follows the constraint proposed in Huang (1984).

Much of the research which suggests that L2 learners do not have access to UG is based on learners' low recognition of subjacency violations. Under our hypothesis, this would be explained by the fact that the learners' grammars did not generate the relevant sentences by movement. However, lack of movement should also be evidenced by the other diagnostics we describe above. We pilot-tested our hypothesis on 27 ESL learners whose native language is Indonesian. Before describing the experiment itself, we will outline some relevant facts in the grammar of Indonesian.

Wh-questions in Indonesian.

Like English, Indonesian has SVO word order. As shown in Table 1 it does not use movement in all the structural configurations where it is required in English. Thus, (1) and (2) below show that wh-questions occur with the wh-word in situ and that movement in simple questions is ungrammatical:

(1) a. *Siapa makan kuih?*
Who eat cake
'Who ate cake?'

b. *Siti makan apa?*
Siti eat what
'What did Siti eat?'

(2) **Apa Siti makan?*
(With the intended meaning: 'What did Siti eat'

There are some types of questions for which it might be argued that movement is involved. Consider, for example, (3) where the object *apa* 'what' appears in sentence-initial position:

(3) *Apa (yang) dimakan Siti?*
What comp pass-eat Siti
'What was eaten by Siti?'

or (4), an indirect question:

(4) *Siapa (yang) kaukira dicium Siti?*
Who comp you-think pass-kiss Siti
'Who do you think was kissed by Siti?'

Several facts indicate however, that neither of these sentences involves movement and that the wh-words *apa* in (3) and *siapa* in (4) are base-generated in sentence-initial position. First, note that for both sentences, crucially the clitic *di-* must attach to the verbs *makan* 'eat' and *-cium* 'kiss', passivizing the sentences and making the wh-words subjects. As a passive, (3) is thus generated with the wh-word *apa* in-situ. As far as sentence (4) is concerned, it might be argued that although *siapa* is base-generated as the subject of *dicium* in the lower clause, it is then moved to the front of the upper clause. However, this argument is countered by evidence that both (3) and (4) in fact represent focused or cleft constructions. Commonly, across languages, such constructions involve a relative (or free relative)-like structure in an equational type sentence as exemplified with the English declarative and interrogative clefts in (5).

(5) a. It was John that ate the cake
b. Who was it that ate the cake?

Arguably, sentences (3) and (4) represent structures parallel to (5b), that is, they consist of a copular clause and a relative clause. The following facts of Indonesian make a strong case for this analysis: As indicated above, both (3) and (4) optionally take *yang*, the relative complementizer, without changing the meaning of the sentences. This strongly suggests that (3) and (4) contain a relative clause but that the relative complementizer is optionally deleted. Evidence for the relative clause also comes from the fact that there is a restriction against object relativization in Indonesian. This explains why (3) and (4) are obligatorily passivized, even when the relative complementizer *yang* does not appear. The lack of a copula is simply explained: Indonesian lacks an overt copula. Thus, the structure of (3) and (4) would parallel (6) and (7), and have the structure shown in (8).

(6) *kuih ini (yang) dimakan Siti*
cake this comp pass-eat Siti
'It was this cake that was eaten by Siti.'

(7) *anak ini (yang) kaukira dicium Siti*
child this comp you-think pass-kiss Siti
'It is this child that you think was kissed by Siti.'

(8) [s [NP] COPULA [NP [s.......Ø..........]]]
+/−WH Ø (relative clause)[2]

The zero copula and optional deletion of the relative complementizer could make it appear as if there were no relative clause in these sentences, i.e., that they are regular wh-questions rather than clefts. However, as shown above, this would fail to explain (a) why passivization is obligatory (i.e. why objects cannot be questioned in this way) and (b) the optional appearance of the relative complementizer *yang* [3] (for more detailed argumentation, see Martohardjono 1988). To summarize, then, wh-in-situ is obligatory for simple questions in Indonesian, and although both object wh-words and lower-clause subject wh-words can appear in sentence-initial position, they can do so only in clefts, where the wh-word is generated in-situ.[4] Thus, in this language wh-questions never involve movement. The apparent wh movement is in fact a function of clefting, for which the argument for no movement in Indonesian is the same as that for relative clauses. There are other languages as well for which what might appears to be Wh movement is actually a subcase of focusing (see for example Gair 1983 for Sinhala, though there, in contrast to Indonesian, the focus is rightward and does involve movement).

Relative Clauses in Indonesian

Martohardjono (1988) argues that relative clauses in Indonesian do not involve movement, and that the relative complementizer *yang* is base-generated in comp. By the theory outlined above, this means that the gap in relative clauses is filled by *pro*. Based on languages such as Chinese, Japanese, German and Portuguese, Huang (1984) argues that for certain types of sentences there is a universal constraint against *pro* in object position.[5] This constraint would provide an explanation for the restriction on object relativization in Indonesian, illustrated in (9):

(9) *anak$_i$ yang Ø$_i$ duduk dibanku.*
child comp e sit LOC-bench
'The child who is sitting on the bench'
**kuihi yang anak makan Ø$_i$*
cake comp child eat e
'The cake that the child ate'

Topics

Indonesian has both gap topics and left-dislocation topics as illustrated in (10) and (11) Interestingly, gap topics obey subjacency, indicating that they are generated by movement, thus differing in this respect from wh-questions and relative clauses. Note also that there is no restriction on topicalizing objects, further strengthening this conclusion.

(10) *anak ini, Siti kemarin tidak lihat Ø*
child this Siti yesterday not see e
'This child, Siti did not see yesterday.'

(11) *anak ini, Siti kemarin tidak melihatnya*
child this Siti not see e AGT-see-him
'This child, Siti did not see him.'

The Experiment

Our primary goal was to determine whether our subjects had movement in their grammars of L2 English, using the movement diagnostics described above. In this paper we report the results of two tests, involving Subjacency and the constraint against pro in object position. In particular, we hypothesized that if there is a point at which learners grammars do not have movement they should allow subjacency violations since it only applies to movement structures, and display a S/O asymmetry in gap constructions, since the gap would be filled by *pro*. On the other hand, if the learners' grammars do instantiate movement, they should obey Subjacency and not display a Subject/Object asymmetry in gap constructions.

Subjects

Subjects were 27 male Indonesian speakers who were studying at a college in Toronto, Ontario. They were on a government sponsored program and had all arrived at the same time in Canada. At the time of testing they had been in Canada for 6 months. All of them had followed the same intensive English course prior to arrival (a six-month-program), and had undergone an ESL placement test upon arrival, administered by the College in Canada.

15 were assessed as "intermediate", 12 as "advanced". Their average age was 27. There was also a control group of 12 native speakers of (American) English.

Test 1

To test whether learners' grammars had the relevant constraint against *pro* in object position, we used an elicited imitation task, which compared wh-constructions with a gap in subject position to those with a gap in object position. Recall that according to the theory, the absence of movement in a grammar forces the gap in these constructions to be filled by *pro*. The constraint against *pro* in object position would then have the effect of rendering sentences with object gaps ungrammatical. We would thus expect more difficulty (i.e. a higher rate of error) in object-gap sentences than in subject-gap sentences). The gap-constructions used were: 2 types of wh-questions (direct and indirect), 2 types of relative clauses (free and regular), 2 types of pseudo-cleft sentences (animate "who" and inanimate "what"). In addition, we used a set of topic constructions: gap topicalization and left dislocation. As mentioned above, in Indonesian topicalization differs from questions and relative clauses in that it is a gap construction which can be generated by movement (cf. Martohardjono 1988). We were interested to see if this fact would have an effect on the L2 grammar, that is, on the way English topicalization structures are treated. Absence of movement in the L2 might be uniform across all structures, or it might be present in some structures only. We reasoned that in the latter situation, absence of movement in the equivalent structure in the L1 might be a contributing factor. We would then expect that topicalization be treated differentially from the other gap-constructions, that is, we would expect that topicalization out of object position be on a par with topicalization out of subject position, since movement would be involved and the constraint against *pro* in object position would not apply here.

Left-dislocation is basically topicalization with a resumptive pronoun, and does not involve movement. An example is given in (12).

(12) This man, I think I know him.

We included these as a comparison to the regular topic constructions, reasoning that it might aid in further assessing the absence or presence of movement in topic constructions for the L2. That is, if left dislocation is easier for the learners to imitate than gap topics, this might be an indication that they prefer constructions without movement in the L2 even under conditions where both the L1 and the L2 allow a functional alternative with movement (i.e. gap topics).

Sentences were controlled for number and type of embedding (see Appendix). The test consisted of two batteries of randomized sentences. Subjects were divided into two groups and were given the batteries in reverse order.

Procedure

The subjects were asked to repeat each sentence as closely as they could. They were told that it was important to complete a sentence once they started repeating, but were allowed 1 repeat presentation. They received a pre-training session in which the vocabulary items used in the test were reviewed and which familiarized them with the task using different typoes of structures of equivalent length. Subjects who were unable to do the training session were disqualified.

Scoring

Changes that did not alter the syntactic structure or meaning of the stimulus sentences were generally scored as correct. For example, in-class substitution of nouns and names (Bill for John, mother for father, etc.), singular for plural, omission of morphemes such as 3rd sg. -s, tense changes ('go' for 'went'), changes in the complementizer ('that' for 'which'), and phonological alterations were not counted as errors. All other changes were scored as incorrect, e.g. incomplete sentences, changing or omitting entire clauses, word substitutions that were not synonymous, changing grammatical relations (e.g. object to subject relativization).

Results for Test 1

Table 2 gives the mean number and percentages of incorrect responses overall, for all WH (movement) sentences with subject gaps and object

Table 2.

		Intermediate	Advanced	Control
a.	Overall errors:			
	mean	16.733 (42%)	6.417 (16%)	0
	SD	4.415	2.575	0
b.	Subject Gap:			
	mean	6.933 (35%)	3.167 (16%)	0
	SD	2.017	1.267	0
c.	Object Gap:			
	mean	9.8 (49%)	3.25 (16%)	0
	SD	2.455	1.603	0

Table 3.

t-tests (two-tailed):

i.	Within-group		
	S/O:	Intermediate	Advanced
		t = -3.494	t=-.141
		p = .0016	p= .8889
ii.	Between-group		
	Overall:	t = -7.162	
		p = .0001	
	Subject:	t = -5.63	
		p = .0001	
	Object:	t = -7.967	
		p = .0001	

gaps for both experimental groups and the control group. Table 3 gives the results of t-tests.

Between-group comparisons show that the two ESL groups differed significantly in their overall performance, as well as in their treatment of subjects gaps and object gaps. Furthermore, both ESL groups differed significantly from the control group overall. Within-group t-tests revealed a difference in the treatment of subject gap sentences vs. object gap sentences, with a significantly higher rate of error for object gaps for the intermediate group, but not for the advanced group.

Discussion

The results of the first test indicate that the groups differed in their overall performance with the advanced group performing significantly better than the intermediate group. This shows that the two groups have different levels of proficiency and generally supports the ESL grouping done by the College. Of interest are the statistics showing the differential treatment of subject vs. object gaps by the intermediate group, but not by the advanced group. The difficulty the intermediate group had with object gaps is explained if we assume that they have pro in the gaps. For the advanced group, the difference in error rate between subject and object gap was minimal (means 3.167 vs. 3.25 , i.e. 16%). This indicates that whatever caused the differential error rate in the grammars of the intermediate group was absent in the advanced group, and supports the hypotheses that (a) the constraint on pro in object position is not in effect for the advanced group, and hence, that (a) the gaps contain variables. The evidence clearly suggests that the grammars differ in the way our hypothesis predicts.

Test 2

We tested for Subjacency in the learners' grammars using a paced Grammaticality Judgment task. Only 9 out of the 15 intermediate subjects and 10 out of the 12 advanced subjects participated in this test which consisted of grammatical and ungrammatical wh-extractions (see appendix).

Table 4.

Results:

	Intermediate	Advanced
Overall correct	66%	91%
Correct/gr	72%	95%
Correct/ung	60%	87%

Table 5.

t-tests

Between-group:

overall correct	t = -5.553,	p = .0001
correct/gr	t = -3.21,	p = .0051
correct/ung	t = -4.359,	p = .0004

Procedure

The test sentences were read out loud to the subjects who also had a written version of the test. They were given 5 seconds to judge each sentence "grammatical" or "ungrammatical". The results are given in Table 4 and t-test results in Table 5.

The results show that both groups performed better on correctly judging grammatical sentences than ungrammatical sentences. The advanced group recognized subjacency violations at a higher rate than the intermediate group and the t-test shows that this difference is statistically significant at $p = .0001$.

Discussion for Tests 1 and 2

A straightforward comparison between test 1 and test 2 cannot be made, since they involved different tasks and scoring procedures. However, the results clearly show that the two groups differed from each other both in terms of treating subject gaps and objects gaps differentially, as well as in terms of recognizing subjacency violations. Insofar as the two phenomena we tested for can be viewed as diagnostics of movement in learners' grammars, we can say that the results suggest differential instantiations of movement by the two groups. This difference is consistent with our hypothesis that the sensitivity of learners' grammars to movement principles varies with the degree to which they have instantiated movement. In particular, the results of the first test are consistent with the hypothesis that the L2 grammars of the intermediate group do not generate the gap structures by movement. This would further explain the depressed rate of recognition of subjacency violations. The results for the advanced group, on the other hand, show no subject/object asymmetry for the gap structures, which is what we would expect from a grammar that instantiates movement. Consequently, their rate of recognition of subjacency violations is higher.

Error Rate by Structure: Intermediate Group

The following table gives the error rates for each type of structure for the intermediate group. As stated earlier, we included the topic constructions to afford a comparison with the wh-constructions.

Table 6.

Error rate in percentages per type of structure (including both subject and object gaps)[6]:

WH-CONSTRUCTIONS:	
Direct Questions:	70%
Indirect Questions:	42%
Rel. Clause (Subject):	45%
Rel. Clause (Object):	40%
Free Rel. Cl. (Subject):	51%
Free Rel. Cl. (Object):	43%
Pseudo-Cleft (who):	60%
Pseudo-Cleft (what):	25%
TOPIC CONSTRUCTIONS	
+MOVEMENT	
Gap-topic:	18%
−MOVEMENT	
Left-Dislocation:	23%

As can be seen in this table, the two topicalization structures, gap topics and left dislocation, have a much lower error rate than the wh-gaps. (The one exception is the low error rate on the pseudo-clefts with what, for which we have no ready explanation at present.) An examination of the LD sentences revealed that errors mainly involved omitting the resumptive pronoun, thus effectively changing it to a gap-topic. Given the marginal status of Left Dislocation, this is not a surprising effect. (Interestingly, this type of error was also the only one committed by the control group. It might thus be tentatively concluded that this type of error did not in fact constitute an error). Note that this effect is the opposite of the possibility we outlined before, that non-movement is generalized across the board for the L2.

The mean error rate for the gap-topics was 18%. Testing for a subject-object asymmetry in the treatment of these structures we did not find a significant difference (p=.7165). Given the low number of sentences per type of structure (4), these results need to be interpreted with caution, yet there is some indication that the topic constructions differed from the rest of the gap-constructions in that they were not responsive to the *pro* constraint we tested for. As mentioned earlier, gap-topics in Indonesian do involve movement (cf. Martohardjono 1988), a fact which might contribute to their differential treatment by the subjects. This then suggests the possibility that the L1 grammar has some influence on the learner's grammar of the L2. That is, those structures which are generated by movement in the L1 may also be generated by movement in the L2.

Our basic hypothesis, stated in the simplest terms, was that the apparent unavailability of UG in second language acquisition, as measured by single-factor experimentation, might in fact be a function not of its unavailability in toto, but of the learner's failure to recognize the applicability of some specific UG principle to a specific L2 structure or structures. We also hypothesized that an interaction with L1 might be a factor in such failure to apply. The results of this pilot project are indeed consistent with and serve to bear out this hypothesis.

On the grammatical judgments of subjacency, the percentage of correct judgments of subjacency violations by the intermediate group accords generally with that found in the experimental studies of other researchers who in fact argue for the unavailability of UG (Schachter 1988, Johnson 1988). There is a clear increase in the scores of the advanced group on this test, which does indeed suggest at the minimum, an increased availability and applicability of the principle of subjacency, since it is difficult to conceive on what basis these judgments might otherwise be made. The case becomes clearer, however, when we take the results of the other experimental tasks into account. Not surprisingly, the intermediate group did far worse overall on the L2 movement structures than the advanced group, but it is the distribution of the errors in terms of gap position that bears most directly on our hypothesis. The advanced group did equally well on subject and object gaps. The intermediate group, however, did much worse on object than on subject gaps. It is at this point that we note that the manner in which the relevant structures are generated in Indonesian, the L1, and the L2 English differ sharply in the empty categories involved, as a reflection of the principles by which they are generated, which in turn leads to a difference in their distribution. The results here are precisely what we would predict if the intermediate learners were applying their L1 principles to these structures; specifically, they are treating the gaps as *pro* rather than as a variable generated by movement. In this case, then, the different scores between L1 and L2 as well as the leveling out between subject and object position indicate that the recognition of movement, and hence the differences in kind and distribution of empty categories, has come into play in the interval: i.e., "clicked in," so to speak. Note, however, that the performance of the intermediate group in terms of differential treatment of subject and object is indeed consistent with UG: it simply invokes the proper UG option for L1, but the wrong one for L2. The "clicking in" thus is not in the appearance of UG, but the correct choice and application of the relevant principles allowed by UG to the relevant structures.

Nor is it the case that the kind of subject-object asymmetry that appeared in the intermediate group is simply some kind of characteristic of L2 acquisition in general. For example, a recent study of Japanese versus Chinese acquirers of English by Flynn and Brown (1988) determined that at a particular stage of advancement, the Chinese did not exhibit such asymmetry, though the Japanese did. Interestingly, we could tentatively conclude that this in fact offers another example for our hypothesis. In the Chinese vs. Japanese case, the same specific factors cannot be at work as with Indonesian, since neither of these languages exhibits subject-object asymmetry in the relevant structures. Rather, the difference appears to involve the ECP together with the fact that canonical government direction differs between the languages. If so, that difference in performance would represent another instance of L1-L2 interaction involving the failure for a time to apply the proper UG principles, though different ones, in L2.

Originally, the topicalized and left-dislocated structures were included in the design as a kind of comparison and control, but in the event, serve to add further confirmation of our hypothesis. On these structures, which are generated similarly in L1 and L2, the intermediate group performed strikingly well. Most importantly, they did not invoke subject-object asymmetry, but quite correctly treated the gaps as traces (variables) from the start. That is, they applied the proper principles, and it seems quite clear that here the L1-L2 parallelism facilitated the necessary recognition. Recall also that the errors that were made were to a great extent not errors at all in terms of allowed L2 output, but rather reflected making the "wrong" choice among options permitted in both L1 and L2. The performance of the intermediate group on this task thus contrasts with that on the other, and strongly supports the conclusion that UG is available to the learner, but that that availability may in at least some instances be masked by failure to recognize and apply the proper specific principle(s) to some structure(s). This conclusion could have been strengthened even further had there been an test for subjacency in topic structures, and this will be included in extending this experimental program beyond the pilot phase.

In short, the results of this pilot study are not only consistent with the initial hypothesis, but serve, as far as they go, to confirm it. The next step will be to broaden the experimental tasks to include the other diagnostics of movement that were listed earlier, to refine the tasks that have been used here, and to broaden the population of subjects. On the basis of our results so far, we are confident that our initial hypothesis will be confirmed, and hopefully, refined.

Afterword

Subsequent to the presentation of our paper, White (to appear) has presented a paper that is in agreement with the general approach we propose for the diagnosis of movement phenomena. She suggests, however, that our particular proposal cannot account for existing SLA data on Subjacency, in particular the results reported by Johnson (1988) and Schachter (1989). She notes that the test sentences used in these studies involved the extraction of objects, e.g.:

*Which test$_i$ don't you know who failed e$_i$

and writes that

> "If the learner has wh-movement, object gaps are wh-traces, subject to Subjacency. If the learner does not have movement, object gaps are prohibited, on Huang's analysis, adopted by Martohardjono and Gair. Therefore, sentences like [these] should be rejected by all learners, regardless of whether they have syntactic wh-movement, as should grammatical wh-questions with object gaps. But what has been found is that L2 learners tend to accept sentences such as these."

While the reasons that learners make the particular kinds of errors they do regarding subjacency or other constraints is certainly not without interest, White's contention is actually beside the point with relation to our paper, which makes no attempt to address such questions. Our essential hypothesis is that learners' errors that appear to violate such UG constraints does not necessarily mean that UC is dead or effete, but that it may simply not apply to particular structures since they have not been analyzed in such a way as to invoke the appropriate constraint. Clearly also, since we dealt with a particular L1 and suggested an analysis of the equivalent structures in that language, there was at least an implicit acceptance of the notion that the particular L1 was not irrelevant in that failure of recognition, though that did not necessarily mean transfer in the usual sense. What would seem most natural to assume here is that the L1 may, on the basis of how it treats particular constructions, either provide or fail to provide a model facilitating or not the acquisition of a particular L2. While this is by no means a startling or implausible assumption, we did not attempt to test it directly.

Looked at in that light, White's comment, and the example she chooses does not bear directly on the validity or lack of it of our claim. To support it, we needed only to show (a) that at an earlier stage, learners made more errors in one condition than in another (i.e., movement versus non-movement), and (b) that that difference was consistent with their lack of recognition, presumably consistent with the nature of their particular L1, that a principle applied. It was not reasonably incumbent upon us to explain why they made the particular errors that they did. As anyone who has spent any considerable time teaching a language knows, the number of devices that a learner may bring to bear in attempting to deal with an L2 are multifarious, nor are they limited to language processes per se, but may indeed be "brute force" operations. With a grammaticality judgement task, the underlying mechanisms are particularly difficult to unravel and identify, as is well known. Thus in the particular example chosen by White, we obviously cannot make claims about the grammars of the subjects in Johnson's or Schachter's study. Nor does our hypothesis help us toward that end, given that there are many possibilities to account for what in this case appears to be a straightforward subjacency violation. It could be, for instance, simply that they have learned that English allows objects to be relativized long distance, and overgeneralize that observation into blanket acceptance, when presented with (for them) complicated examples overtaxing their processing capabilities. Note, however, that this would be perfectly consistent with our claim that UG may still be available, but that the learners may not, at one stage, recognize that particular principles apply (in this case, that movement is involved), so that UG does not "click in". Looked at in that way, examples such as those that White adduces, along with her observation that principles seem to be ignored, are not inconsistent with our hypothesis. Rather, when taken together with the fact that there is indeed subsequent recognition of those principles, as evidenced by the performance of advanced students, they can in fact be taken to support it.

Notes

*We would like to thank Barbara Lust, Suzanne Flynn, Wayne Harbert, Jim Huang, and Wayne O'Neil, for comments and discussion along with all of those who offered comments or questions at the Conference itself and the Spring 1989 seminar on UG and Second Language Acquisition at MIT at which a version of this paper was presented. The usual disclaimers apply.

1. For a different interpretation of Schachter's result, see Eubank (1989).

2. We do not enter here into the strucure of free relatives in Indonesian. Whether they are internally headed or have an external phonologically null head are interesting questions, but go beyond the scope of this paper which requires only that they be identifiable.

3. In some dialects, including that of GM, omission of the *yang* is not allowed, making the cleft/non-cleft distinction even more clear.

4. A similar phenomenon occurs in Nicaraguan English Creole (O'Neill p.c.).

5. There is an interesting debate in the linguistic literature regarding the universality of this constraint, which for obvious reasons we cannot go into here. The reader is referred to Huang (1984), Xu and Langendoen (1985) and Huang (1987). For a parameterized version of Huang's analysis, see Cole (1987).

6. For both types of relative clauses, there was some difference in performance depending on whether the entire relative complex was in subject or object position in the matrix clause. The error rates were Rel Clause: Subject 45%, Object 40%; Free relatives: Subject 51%, Object 43%. The subjects thus performed better in matrix object position, but here, of course, a difference in gaps is not involved, since we are dealing only with the external structural position of the relative complex.

References

Bley-Vroman, Robert. 1989. "What is the Logical Problem of Foreign Language Learning?". *Linguistic Perspectives on Second Language Acquisition*. ed. by S. Gass and J. Schachter, 41-68. Cambridge: Cambridge University Press.

Bley-Vroman, Robert, Sascha Felix and Georgette Ioup. Forthcoming. "The Accessibility of Universal Grammar in Adult Language Learning". To appear in *Studies in Second Language Acquisition*.

Chomsky, Noam. 1982. *Some Concepts and Consequences of the Theory of Government and Binding*. (Linguistic Inquiry Monograph 6). Cambridge, MA: MIT Press.

Clahsen, Harald and Pieter Muysken. 1986. "The Availability of Universal Grammar to Adult and Child Learners: A study of the Acquisition of German Word Order". *Second Language Research* 2.93-119.

Cole, Peter. 1987. "Null Objects in Universal Grammar". *Linguistic Inquiry* 18.597-612.

Corder, S.P. 1967. "The Significance of Learners' Errors". *International Review of Applied Linguistics* 5.161-70.

Eubank, Lynn. 1989. "Testing a Revised Universal". Mimeographed ms. University of Hawai'i at Manoa.

Flynn, Suzanne. 1984. "A Universal in L2 Acquisition Based on a PBD Typology". *Universals of Second Language Acquisition* ed. by Fred Eckman, Lawrence Bell and Diane Nelson, 75-87. Rowley, MA: Newbury House.

Flynn, Suzanne. 1987. *A Parameter-setting Model of L2 Acquisition*. Dordrecht: D. Reidel Publishing Company.

Flynn, Suzanne. 1988. "Nature of Development in L2 Acquisition and Implications for Theories of Language Acquisition in General". Flynn and O'Neil 1988.76-89.

Flynn, Suzanne and Brown. 1988. "Three Patterns of Development in Adult Second Language Learning". M.S., M.I.T.

Flynn, Suzanne and Wayne O'Neil, eds. 1988. *Linguistic Theory in Second Language Acquisition*. Dordrecht: Kluwer Academic Publishers.

Gair, James W. 1983. "Non-configurationality, Movement, and Sinhala Focus". Paper delivered at the Linguistics Association of Great Britain. March 1983 Meeting.

Huang, C.T.J. 1980. "Topicalization and Relativization in Chinese". Mimeographed manuscript, MIT.

Huang, C.T.J. 1984. "On the Distribution and Reference of Empty Pronouns". *Linguistic Inquiry* 15.531-74.

Jaeggli, Osvaldo and Ken Safir. 1989. "The Null Subject Parameter and Parametric Theory". *The Null Subject Parameter* ed. by Osvaldo Jaeggli and Ken Safir, 1-44. Dordrecht: D. Reidel Publishing Company.

Johnson, Jacqueline S. 1988. *Critical period effects on universal properties of language: The status of subjacency in the acquisition of a second language*. Unpublished Ph. D. dissertation, University of Illinois at Urbana-Champaign.

Kaswanti Purwo, B. 1981. Kata Yang Sebagai Pengetat. *Majalah Pembinaan Bahasa Indonesia* IV/3.175-85.

Liceras, Juana. 1989. "L2 Learnability: Delimiting the Domain of Core Grammar as Distinct from the Marked Periphery". Flynn and O'Neil 1988.199-224.

Martohardjono, G. 1988. Yang-phrases in Indonesian. Mimeographed ms. Cornell University.

Raposo, Eduardo. 1986. *On the Null Object in European Portuguese: Studies in Romance Linguistics*. Dordrecht: Foris.

Ritchie, William. 1978. "The Right Roof Constraint in an Adult-acquired Language". *Second Language Acquisition Research* ed. by W. Ritchie, 33-63. New York: Academic Press.

Schachter, Jacquelyn. 1988.

Schachter, Jacquelyn. 1990. "On the Issue of Completeness in Second Language Acquisition". *Second Language Research* 6.93-124.

Selinker, Larry. 1972. Interlanguage. *International Review of Applied Linguistics* 10.209-31.

Taraldsen, T. 1978. "On the NIC, Vacuous Application and the That-trace Filter". Mimeographed manuscript, MIT.

White, Lydia. 1986. "Implications of Parametric Variation for Adult Second Language Acquisition: An Investigation of the "Pro-drop" Parameter". *Experimental Approaches to Second Language Acquisition* ed. by V. Cook. Oxford: Pergamon Press.

White, Lydia. To appear. "Subjacency Relations and Empty Categories in Second Language Acquisition. *Island Constraints: Theory, Processing and Acquisition*. ed. by H. Goodluck and M. Rochemont. Dordrecht: Kluwer.

Appendix

Test 1 sample sentences:

Indirect Question:
 Subject extraction:
  Sue asked John what books were on sale at the University bookstore.

 Object extraction:
  Before he left, Bill told Sue what museums she should visit in Paris.

Direct Question:
 Subject extraction:
  What country did you say has won the most medals in the Olympics?

 Object extraction:
  What does Mary think her mother will say when she tells her about John?

Relative Clause in subject position:
 Subject gap:
  The books which were on sale today were on the bestseller's list last year.

 Object gap:
  The new car which Sue bought for her mother was quite expensive.

Relative Clause in object position
 Subject gap:
  John bought the books which were on sale at the University bookstore.

 Object gap:
  Bill is eating the apples which his wife bought at the market.

Free Relative in subject position
 Subject gap:
  Mary thinks that what is in today's newspaper is very interesting.

 Object gap:
  I hope what we ordered from that store last month will arrive soon.

Free Relative in object position
 Object gap:
  I read in a book that wild animals always eat what they catch.

 Subject gap:
  When John took the money, he did what he thought was right.

Pseudo-Cleft, What
 Subject:
  In this country, what makes people happy is to have money.

 Object:
  Before Bill died, what he wanted was to see his child.

Pseudo-Cleft, Who
Subject:
Sue says that who worries her is her son.

Object:
Mary thinks that who I saw was her husband.

Topicalization
Subject:
Japanese food, Bill says is much too expensive in this city.

Object:
Pizza, I think John said he likes with mushrooms and cheese.

Left Dislocation
Subject:
Elizabeth Taylor, I think she lives in a mansion in California.

Object:
This movie, Bill said he watched it three times in a row.

Test 2:

Grammatical wh-extraction:
What did the doctor say he thought should be done for John?

Ungrammatical wh-extraction:
*Who did you read the news had won the elections yesterday?

Parameter-resetting in Second Language Acquisition:

A Study of Adult Spanish and Vietnamese Learners of English

Elizabeth Platt
Florida State University

Introduction

The present debate in second language acquisition (SLA) research in the psycholinguistic perspective centers on the issue of whether to best characterize knowledge of the second language (L2) with respect to 1) the contribution of general cognitive characteristics of the learner or 2) the specific contribution of the linguistic structure. The latter approach has been taken in a comparative study of adult learners of English representing typologically different languages, Spanish and Vietnamese. As linguistic theory in the generative framework has become a theory of innate constraints on syntactic representations as opposed to one of rule generation, it has attracted renewed interest for language acquisition researchers. Claims made within the principles and parameters framework specifically define the nature of the acquisition process, and are empirically verifiable. While a proper theory of SLA will ultimately stipulate the relationship between cognitive and linguistic structures, studies such as the present one attempt to delineate the domain of the grammar and to show its impact on the development of particular grammatical structures.

The object studied was the null subject phenomenon, superficially similar in Spanish and Vietnamese, but with different underlying identification and licensing principles. The hypotheses were derived from Hyams' (1986) claim that English-speaking children begin thinking that English is an agreement language, allowing null subjects, or pro-drop. When they notice that their language requires non-thematic subjects (*it*, *there*) in tensed clauses, they restructure the early stage grammar, consistent with English, a non-pro-drop language. Hyams' (1986) claims for first language acquisition were substantiated by the work of Hilles (1986) who found in a longitudinal study that one Spanish-speaking 12 year-old apparently acquired these theoretically-related features simultaneously.

The present cross-sectional study tested whether Spanish-speaking adult learners would show a similar pattern, and whether Vietnamese speakers would perform likewise. However, the findings of this study were that on a grammatical judgment task Spanish speakers performed less well on items testing presence or absence of the English obligatory subject with respect to auxiliaries, while the Vietnamese speakers demonstrated a similar pattern of mastery for both subjects and auxiliaries. The similar orders of difficulty attained by the Vietnamese speakers of NP features and AUX features demonstrates that the grammatical knowledge represented as NP and AUX constructs operationalized in the task is uniform in complexity. That Spanish speakers failed to show as strong a relationship between the variables as the Vietnamese suggests a possible inhibitory factor in SLA. That factor is arguably linked to agreement; Spanish speakers assume English to be an agreement language. Only after they learn that null referential subjects are not identified, and that null expletives are not licensed, can Spanish speakers be said to have reset the parameter associated with pro-drop, or null subjects.

The paper is organized as follows: in the first section the theoretical issues concerning the null subject phenomena are discussed, followed by a statement of the hypotheses and predictions. The design and results are presented next, with discussion and concluding remarks.

Theoretical Issues: Null Subjects

The theory for this study is the principles and parameters approach (Chomsky 1981, 1986), one widely taken in recent SLA studies (see White 1984; Cook 1985; Flynn and O'Neil 1988). This approach posits a set of highly constrained principles which interact to produce abstractly-related syntactic phenomena, and which are fixed with experience of the first language. This fixing is called parameter setting, resetting in SLA. Sanctioning of null nominal elements follows from the operation of several principles, among them the projection principle, binding and government. The projection principle states that representations are uniform across levels. Thus, to show movement, the principles and parameters theory posits the existence of traces, one type of null element. Binding in the larger sense pertains to the coreference of both overt and null elements within the sentence (Rizzi 1986). Government is a central unifying concept of UG which pertains to the relationship of lexical or functional heads and the elements within the maximal projection, or highest phrasal level, of the head (Aoun and Sportiche 1983; Hyams 1986).

Among the several functions of government is the sanctioning of the absence of elements from their canonical positions, and the constraining of movement from certain positions in a sentence. Pronominals may be null in several environments in languages, and they are of several types, just as lexical NPs are. While traces relate to moved elements, PRO and *pro* are base-generated. PRO is the null NP occupying the position of subject of a non-tensed clause, either controlled by a superordinate clause NP or assigned an arbitrary reading. PRO is a base-generated element lacking a governing category, a situation which follows from PRO's status as both anaphor and pronominal. Sentence (1) illustrates this contradiction.

(1) I like PRO to play baseball.

In the example PRO is anaphoric since it is coindexed with the higher clause subject, pronominal in that it acts as the subject of the lower clause. Such a situation being vacuous creates an environment for non-government. The other null NP is *pro*, a base-generated pronominal which usually occurs in languages either by agreement as in Spanish and Italian (2), or by some other means as in the case of Chinese and Vietnamese (3).

(2) *pro vengo a las siete.*
(I) am coming at seven.

(3) *pro có thê đi học được*
(One) can go to school.

Specification of the means to accomplish identification and licensing for null elements in each language type, and of the parameter or parameter settings associated with empty categories, are ongoing issues in theoretical linguistics (Huang 1984a,b; Adams 1987; Rizzi 1986; Cole 1987; Jaeggli and Hyams 1987; Hermon and Yoon 1989). Principles by which *pro* can be identified and licensed are discussed in the next two sections. This study focuses on the problem of how adult learners of English speaking null subject languages as L1, Spanish or Vietnamese, come to know that their L2 does not permit null subjects. Thus, it is important to know why some languages sanction them, and why others do not, and to distinguish between the principles under which subjects can be omitted in languages so dissimilar as Spanish and Vietnamese.

Null Subjects in Spanish

In languages like Spanish and Italian agreement suffixes on verbs *identify* null subjects. Identification pertains to person, number and gender features encoded on the verb which identify, but might not uniquely specify, the referent with which they are coindexed. *Licensing* is provided by some putative property of languages such as morphological uniformity (Jaeggli and Hyams 1987), head direction assignment (Adams 1987) or by a governing and a case-assigning head, a licensing independent of identification by feature specification (Rizzi 1986). Languages like Spanish and Italian contain agreement (AGR) in INFL, and are characterized by the following cluster of properties: a) missing subjects, b) free inversion in simple sentences, c) "long *wh-* movement" of subject, d) empty resumptive pronouns in embedded clauses, and e) apparent violations of the *that-* trace filter (Chomsky, 1981). Later analyses have posited the inclusion of slightly different clusters of properties. This version of the Pro(nominal)-drop Parameter has been replaced by newer versions positing underlying relationships of other clusters of properties, and the relevant parameter is labelled the Null Subject Parameter. By any definition of the parameter, languages either do, or do not, allow null subjects.

The description of the parameter used in this study is an analysis which relates null subjects and certain features of the auxiliary system directly to the properties of AGR in INFL (Hyams 1986). This analysis was intended to explain certain facts of the acquisition of English by young children. Hyams observed that English-speaking children pass through a stage where their speech is characterized by 1) the occurrence of both subjectless sentences and sentences with subjects, 2) the absence of expletives, and 3) the absence of auxiliaries. The first two properties of child language are also characteristic of Spanish, the parameter setting of which English-speaking youngsters are assumed to begin, by this account. This analysis assumes that heads govern complements, and some elements within those complements. INFL as the head of the sentence governs and assigns nominative case to the subject. The structure of INFL for adult Spanish and for the initial stage grammar of children is shown in (A), where AGR heads INFL. AGR is the abstract element which coindexes with person and number features on the verb suffix, thus identifying pro. According to Rizzi (1982), the features of AGR (person and number) are pronominal, and as such assign both case and theta-roles to *pro*, and properly govern the null subject. Hyams extended Rizzi's analysis to claim that AGR=PRO, arguing as follows: When AGR heads INFL, AUX surfaces in VP, thus has no sister dominated by INFL. Since AGR has no sister, the implication is that AUX must not be in INFL where it would govern AGR. Thus, being ungoverned, AGR must be PRO.

```
(A)          INFL
            /    \
AGR/PRO       (AUX)
```

Hyams' (1986) claim is that when children notice unstressed referential pronouns and/or expletives occurring in English, the restructuring of the initial state grammar is triggered. Restructuring produces the adult grammar of English in which AUX heads INFL, thus is no longer a constituent of VP. When Aux moves into INFL, AGR can no longer be PRO, as shown in (B).

```
(B)          INFL
            /    \
AG =/PRO      AUX
```

Hyams (1986) favors an explanation whereby triggering is accomplished by the acquisition of expletives, because they are obligatorily present in English, null in Spanish. Since the occurrence of overt referential pronouns is regulated by pragmatic rather than syntactic considerations in Spanish, the initial "language," it is less likely that their obligatory presence in English sentences is salient to the child learner. While this interesting analysis has been challenged, both by its own author (Hyams 1987) and others (Guilfoyle 1984; LeBeaux 1987), the observations about child language must still be explained, and the relationship between null subjects and the consequences of an agreement system is still valid. These consequences are specified in the section on auxiliaries.

Null Subjects in Vietnamese

In languages like Vietnamese arguments may be deleted freely, pragmatic as well as syntactic considerations determining when NPs may be null

(Pingkarawat 1989). The most extensive analysis of null NPs in languages of this type in the literature is that of Huang (1984a,b) who accounts for the distribution and referencing of null nominal elements by the operation of several identifying principles and an additional device: the disjoint reference rule (DJR), the generalized control rule (GCR), and the empty topic operator. The DJR states that *pro*, being pronominal, must not be coindexed with any c-commanding element in its governing category, since pronominals must by Binding Theory be free in their governing category. The GCR is stated as in (4).

(4) An empty pronominal is controlled in its control domain (if it has one). (p. 193)

"Control domain" entails the notions of c-commanding NP and accessible SUBJECT. Huang accepts only one true pronominal in Chinese, that being subject to the rule of control generalized to deal with both PRO and *pro* (Huang 1989). Lehman and Pingkarawat (1985), and Pingkarawat (1989) also argue for a single base-generated pronominal in Thai and Burmese. In sentences (2) and (3) in Chinese the GCR identifies both a PRO and a *pro* respectively (recall that PRO is the ungoverned element, having both pronominal and anaphoric properties in languages such as English). In the sentences below *e* is used to denote any empty category: PRO, *pro* or variable.

(5) *Zhangsan$_i$ shefa e$_i$ bangmang wo*
Zhangsan try e help I
'Zhangsan tries to help me.'

(6) *Zhangsan$_i$ shuo [e$_{i,j}$ bu renshi Lisi]*
Zhangsan say [e not know Lisi]
'Zhangsan says he doesn't know Lisi.'

The notion that an empty topic operator (Huang 1984a,b) is present in languages like Chinese follows from the interaction of the GCR and the DJR. If a null object were *pro*, it would be required by the GCR to be coindexed with its clausemate subject, the closest nominal element. But since such coindexing would violate the DJR, the null object can only be coindexed with a non-c-commanding NP. Such NPs are found only in non-argument positions like the topic position, and null objects can only be variables. Like *wh-* elements, variables are traces, coindexed with the operator to which they are bound. This operator can also identify null NPs in subject position.

As for licensing of null subjects in Chinese, Huang (1984a) claims that since they can be null, they must therefore be properly governed by INFL. Proper government by INFL extends also to the topic, which can also be null.[1]

Strong arguments can be made for using Huang's analysis of Chinese for Vietnamese data; the null subject and object in sentence (7) could be accounted for by the postulation of an empty topic operator containing two topics.[2]

(7) *e Khoĝng neĝn gọi e vì bà ấy mẹt lắm.*
e not should call e because she tired very
'One/you should not call her because she is very tired.'

However, one important factor in Vietnamese, like other widely-observed features of languages of the region, is that null arguments may be non-specific or arbitrary in reference (Lehman and Pingkarawat 1985). This means that they do not have to be identified, usually considered a major criterion in sanctioning null subjects in other languages (Jaeggli and Hyams 1987). For example, sentence (7) could have an arbitrary reading for the subject, namely *one*. Sentences (8) and (9) illustrate the pervasiveness of the arbitrary reading for the null subject. Neither a topic nor the GCR can account for instances of the null nominal elements therein. The most remarkable cases are those in which neither subject in a complex construction has a specific referent, but the references cannot be to the same person or entity. In (8) the subject of the first clause is the leaver, of the second, the one left. In (9) the upstairs clause subject is the item purchased; in the lower it is the buyer, though both are non-specific entities. The *e* in the examples represents the empty category. The sentences are from Hoa (1966).

(8) *Vậy thì e đi tức là e chêt trong lóng một chút.*
Whenever e go means e die in heart a little.
"Whenever a love is gone, one loses a part of his heart."

(9) *Mà e rẻ hơn, thì e cũng phải có tiền.*
Even though e cheap more, so e also must have money
"Even though something is cheaper, one still needs money."

The consequences of there being no strong requirement for the identification of null pronominals in Vietnamese are either 1) that learners of a language like English will have considerable difficulty learning where NPs are obligatory, or 2) that they will notice quite early that subjects are required in English, since positive evidence exists in the form of expletives, indicating that tensed clauses must have overt subjects. One problem with the second option is that since Vietnamese lacks a tense and auxiliary system with the same systematic properties found in INFL in Spanish and English, Vietnamese-speaking learners of English should have considerable difficulty distinguishing when tensing conditions are met. However, since this study did not manipulate tensing, no such claim could be tested.

Auxiliaries

According to Hyams, the restructuring of the early stage grammar has consequences for the auxiliary system, mainly that it appears in AUX rather than VP. For this study the construct "auxiliary knowledge" was operationalized in two ways, 1) the presence of modals or forms of *be* and 2) the position of the auxiliary with respect to *not*. (Full auxiliary knowledge is also dependent on the use of its elements with appropriate verb tense or aspect forms, although this knowledge is not implied in the hypotheses stated in the next section.) Development of the auxiliary system in English by young children is a gradual process, with auxiliaries being absent during the optional subject stage (Bloom 1970). While for children in this stage the acquisition of common modals such as *can* and *will* precedes that of less common ones (Major, 1974), forms of *be* are imitated less in elicitation tasks than modals (Brown and Fraser, 1964). Hyams (1986) claimed that unanalyzed auxiliaries are filtered out by the child's grammar during this period. Children acquire the correct placement of negating elements such as *not* in the following order — 1) sentence negation, 2) negation in VP and 3) negation intervening between AUX and VP (Bellugi 1967). By Hyams' analysis, children demonstrate that AUX has moved into INFL when they reach this last stage. For the purposes of this study it was hypothesized that adult Spanish speakers learning English would achieve this stage coincidental with the onset of obligatory subjects.

Since AUX is in VP in Spanish, the consequences are that modals behave like main verbs, taking the full range of suffixes, but as in English they occur with the infinitival forms of the main verb. Forms of *estar*, *be*, are also fully inflected, as they are in English, and occur with verbs having aspectual suffixes such as *-ando*, *ing*, and its allomorphs. Vietnamese lacks the systematic properties of auxiliaries found in European languages. A few pre-verbal particles optionally express temporal, aspectual or modal notions, although the position of these elements is not fixed. There is no agreement, there being no suffixation in the language. English has a "morphologically non-uniform" auxiliary system (Jaeggli and Hyams 1987), meaning that both inflected and uninflected verb forms occur in the language. Further, the marking of tense and/or agreement occurs either in INFL on the auxiliary or in VP on the verb, depending on whether or not the utterance is declarative. For youngsters learning English the acquisition of this system is a slower process than is the acquisition of the Italian system for young Italian learners (Hyams 1986).

Most students of English as a second language experience difficulty mastering the system. However, in the experience of this researcher, speakers of Vietnamese are particularly susceptible to errors in the acquisition of this system. Vietnamese auxiliaries lack the systematic properties of auxiliaries found in Indo-European languages. A few pre-verbal particles optionally express tense, aspect and mode. These may be considered AUX, although some of these particles may also occur as main verbs. The language is essentially monosyllabic, allowing no encoding of nominal information on the verb. Temporality in Vietnamese is indicated by means of sentence-initial adverbs. Following are examples of tense, aspect and modal particles. They ordinarily appear before the verb as in (10), and before particles of negation as in (11). These sentences were used to elicit data from Vietnamese-speaking consultants, and were judged grammatical.

(10) Cô phải *ăn cơm.*
You must eat rice

(11) *Ông ấy sẽ không mua ào quán rẻ.*
He fut not buy clothes cheap

However, the position of these auxiliary-like elements is not fixed. When *được* has the meaning 'get the opportunity' (a sort of positive passive meaning), it appears before the verb as in (12). When it means *be able* it appears after it as in (13). *Be able* can also be expressed with *có thể* before the verb and *được* optionally after it as in example (14). Another particle, *nên* may appear before the negative, as in (15). This suggests that the word order of negative and auxiliaries with respect to the verb is not grammatically stable as it is in English.

(12) *Anh tôi được đi Cưu Kim Sơn.*
Brother my get opportunity go San Francisco

(13) *Anh tôi chạy không được.*
Brother my run not able

(14) *Chúng tôi có thể di học được*
We have ability go school able

(15) *Không nên gọi vì bà ấy mẹt lắm.*
Not should call because she tired very
"(We) should not call (her) because she is very tired."

The point to be made in this discussion of auxiliaries, and the earlier discussion of null subjects in Vietnamese, has been to demonstrate a problem using Huang's analysis of Chinese for this language. While he claims that INFL government sanctions null subjects, there is no apparent relationship between tense, aspect and modal marking, and the presence or absence of subjects. Thus, there should be no connection among these elements as Vietnamese speakers reset the parameter as they learn English.

SLA Studies of the Null Subject

SLA studies of the null subject from within the GB framework have been reported by White (1985), Hilles (1986) and Phinney (1987). The effects of the resetting of the relevant parameter in SLA have been viewed using a variety of syntactic analyses and data collection techniques. Each has found support for the effects of parametrically-related factors in the acquisition of English by Spanish speakers. A comparative study of adult native speakers of Spanish and of French was reported by White (1985) who used a grammatical judgment task to test the negative setting of the pro-drop parameter, as represented by both French and English. As in the present study, White attempted to determine whether features associated with this parameter were manifested in the performance of Spanish speakers, although she tested features related under the earlier pro-drop analysis (Chomsky, 1981), namely null subjects, *that*-trace effects and subject inversion. Speakers of French were predicted to judge accurately the grammaticality of sentences testing these features, the Spanish speakers less so. While both L1 groups performed similarly on sentences testing *that*-trace effects and subject inversion, the French speakers rejected significantly more items with null subjects than the Spanish speakers, as White had predicted. Thus, she claimed support for a parameter-resetting model.

Hilles tested Hyams' (1986) FLA claims using longitudinal data from a 12 year-old Spanish speaker learning English. In support of Hyams, Hilles found that markedly more frequent use of obligatory referential pronouns and auxiliaries appeared in the child's data samples about the same time that expletives began being used spontaneously. This pattern lead Hilles to conclude that expletive acquisition may indeed trigger the restructuring of the grammar, signalling a resetting of the parameter.

Phinney (1987) documented the order of acquisition of the English obligatory subject by analyzing compositions produced by adult native speakers of Spanish and of English. Using this cross-linguistic study Phinney attempted to establish that pro-drop was the unmarked setting of the parameter. She argued that her findings showed that since English speakers learned to drop pronouns more frequently than Spanish speakers supplied them, English was the marked language on this parameter. Additionally, she found that referential pronouns occurred in obligatory contexts most frequently, followed by non-referential and expletive pronouns. These findings pose a problem for a hypothesis based on the postulation of an expletive trigger, because expletives certainly could not have been learned prior to referential pronouns if they were used less frequently. Phinney argued that her findings were predicted by the analysis of Suñer (1982) who posited that in languages like Spanish a difference exists between *pro* and *ex*, the empty category representing the null expletive. According to Suñer, *ex* does not even receive a d-structure interpretation. Thus, as Phinney claimed, it should be much more difficult to learn that these elements must be overt in a non-pro-drop language like English.

Hypotheses

Consistent with Hyams' (1986) claim for English acquisition by children and with the findings of Hilles (1986) in her longitudinal study of a Spanish speaker learning English, the hypotheses for this study are stated as follows:

1. Spanish speakers learning English will demonstrate a relationship of overall NP and AUX variables consistent with the developmental phenomena observed for children learning English as their first language. This relationship will be indicated by means of a high correlation between AUX and NP variables scores for all learners.
2. The Spanish speakers will demonstrate an order of mastery in which expletives reach criterion before auxiliaries.

3. The L1 Vietnamese-speaking learners of English will not demonstrate a relationship of the NP and AUX variables. This lack of relationship will be manifested as lower correlations of the NP and AUX variables than those achieved by the Spanish speakers.
4. The Vietnamese-speaking learners will not demonstrate an order of mastery in which expletives reach criterion before auxiliaries.

When the child notices that unstressed referential pronouns and/or expletives are required, s/he restructures the early stage grammar. This restructuring not only involves the acquisition of the obligatory subject in non-coordinate tensed clauses, but also has consequences for the auxiliary system. (This term is operationally defined in the next section.) As has been demonstrated in the previous section, the reason for this restructuring relates to the setting of a parameter which allows lexical material in AUX, but disallows null subjects. This first hypothesis is a weak statement of the Hyams (1986) claim, for although it predicts a relationship, it does not predict an ordered one. A stronger claim is derivable from Hyams' analysis, namely that when Spanish-speaking learners notice and begin using expletives, they will move AUX into INFL. As the triggering data, expletives should precede a rapid acquisition of auxiliary information, as expressed in the second hypothesis.

Since there is no relationship of NP and AUX in Vietnamese, speakers of that language are not expected to perform like the Spanish speakers. While Vietnamese permits null subjects, it does not have the same identification and licensing principles as Spanish. In the absence of a relationship, no particular order of mastery of the NP and AUX variables tested in this study is hypothesized. Thus, hypotheses (3) and (4) are the weak and strong hypotheses respectively for the Vietnamese speakers.

While these hypotheses imply L2 differences between the two L1 groups, they go beyond stating that L1 effects will be found in L2. Consistent with predictions from the principles and parameters framework, they state a relationship between two aspects of the language which, though superficially unrelated, are related at an abstract level. If some kind of relationship can be found to hold between the two types of knowledge for the Spanish speakers, then the parameter-setting framework is legitimized as at least a partial model of learner grammars.

Predictions of the four hypotheses, which are in turn based on the Hyams (1986) analysis, provide a test of the parameter-setting framework.

These having been specified, two alternative theories may also be tested using the design of this study. If surface level transfer (Lado 1983) is at work, then Vietnamese- and Spanish-speaking subjects should perform similarly on the items testing the presence or absence of referential and expletive subjects, the environments for potential subject deletion in tensed clauses being similar in the two languages. However, since auxiliaries are quite different for the two languages, performance on the items testing auxiliaries should be different, with the Spanish speakers outperforming the Vietnamese. On the other hand, if complexity of the target language is the primary motivating factor in SLA, then a cross-sectional study should produce a pattern of results showing improvement in performance across the proficiency levels, the L1 groups performing equivalently on both NP and AUX variables.

Method

Subject Selection

The study reported in this paper used data from 50 Spanish speakers and 32 Vietnamese speakers, who ranged from low intermediate to advanced levels of English proficiency. Subjects sought were as similar as possible on several selection variables. First, since age has been found to produce significant differences in acquisition studies, subjects between 15 and 25 at the onset of acquisition were used. According to studies of late learners of morphology in American Sign Language (Newport and Supalla forthcoming), of language-specific morphology of English (Johnson and Newport 1989) and of the subjacency principle (Johnson 1988), learners in their mid-teens and above have been found not to perform at the level of native speakers on tests of grammatical judgment. The upper age limit was selected to make the age group homogeneous. Second, to make educational experience comparable, subjects should have completed between 10 and 16 years of school. Third, since the test was administered in both written and taped form, subjects had to be able to read and write English, and to recognize all vocabulary items on the task. Fourth, to control possible effects of other languages, only monolingual subjects were sought. Subjects having been selected according to these criteria, they were also compared in terms of overall proficiency as measured by means of a 45-item multiple choice test,

Table 1. Performance on the Proficiency Measure by L1 and Level

	L1	N	Mean	SD	Var	T	df	P
Low level	S	16	14.3	3.96	equal	1.09	24	.29
	V	10	12.6	3.83				
Middle level	S	22	23.3	2.34	equal	.55	31	.58
	V	11	22.8	2.68				
High level	S	12	32.3	4.10	equal	-0.74	21	.46
	V	11	33.6	4.34				
Total	S	50	22.6	7.53	uneq	-0.38	56	.71
	V	32	23.3	9.36				

items for which were taken from the placement profile of the Intensive English Institute at the University of Illinois. Items tested morphological marking, word order and grammatical morpheme choice. Subjects were divided into three groups on the basis of performance on this test. Table 1 shows the number of subjects in each proficiency level by L1 group. Means are number correct out of 45.

Finally, as found in interviews, subject groups were comparable in terms of the amount of time they had spent in the United States, of attitudes toward L1 and L2, and of motivation to achieve and maintain proficiency in both languages. Subjects were tested in high school, college and agency settings in the cities of Urbana and Chicago, Illinois, and Lincoln, Nebraska.

Instrument: Grammatical Judgment Task

A grammatical judgment task (GJT) was the main task of the study. The 96-item task assessed knowledge of the features associated with the English setting of the null subject parameter. The items were presented simultaneously in both written and audio-recorded form to all subjects to avoid potential perceptual bias. Subjects responded 'yes' or 'no' to each item, having been told in the instructions to attend to forms of words, order of constituents and words left out. The instrument was designed so that there were an equal number of correct and incorrect responses, and an equal number of each of the twelve variable types described below. As shown in the examples, target sentences (in bold) were preceded by lead sentences, which disambiguated the referent in the instances where presence or absence of referential pronouns was being tested, and made all the other items uniform with them. Six NP (noun phrase) variables tested the presence or absence of subject pronouns: 1) singular and 2) plural referential pronouns, 3) weather *it*, 4) raising *it*, and 5) singular and 6) plural subjects with *there* preposed. Six AUX (auxiliary) variables tested auxiliary knowledge: the presence or absence of 8) *be* or 9) modals, the position of *not* with respect to 10) *be* or 11) modals, and the marking of 11) tense or 12) aspect on the verb. In all there were eight of each of the twelve types.

Sentences in Grammatical Judgment Task

Presence or absence of referential pronoun

1. Singular

   One day my sister was walking to school. **All of a sudden (she) saw a small bird near the bushes.**

2. Plural

   For five hundred years the church bells rang every hour. **After lightning hit them, (they) did not ring again.**

Presence or absence of *it*

3. Weather *it*

   Last week everyone enjoyed the good weather. **On Monday (it) was very warm outside.**

4. Raising *it*

   I like to go out in my car on Sundays. **When I drive up the hill, (it) is possible to see far below me.**

Presence or absence of *there*

5. Singular

   Yesterday I heard a noise from a tree. **When I looked up, (there) was a cat on a branch in the tree.**

6. Plural

   My grandmother had a beautiful home. **A long time ago (there) were many big plants in her living room.**

Presence or absence of auxiliary

7. *Be*

   Last summer we saw a water show in Florida. **When we went in, some fish (were) jumping out of the water.**

8. Modal

   Tomorrow there is a party in my uncle's office. **For the party he (will) wear a white shirt with a jacket.**

Position of auxiliary with respect to the position of *not*

9. *Be*

These days our old dog is feeling sick. **This evening he (not) is (not) eating his food.**

10. Modal

My mother left her keys at the church. **Because she has no keys, she (not) can (not) open her car.**

Presence or absence of verb marking with marked auxiliary

11. *Be*

Yesterday morning I asked my husband about the money. **But when I talked to him, he was not listen(ing).**

12. Modal

Somebody put a dead rat in the kitchen. **Because the room smelled bad, my sister would not enter(ed) it.**

Results

Correlational Analyses

Several types of statistical analyses were used to test the four hypotheses listed in the previous section. As a preliminary test of the first and third hypotheses, correlational analyses were run using the data of all the subjects. Results of these analyses supported the first but challenged the third hypotheses, because they determined a higher correlation of the variables for the Vietnamese than for the Spanish speakers (.80 and .69 respectively with a probability of less than .0001 for both correlations occurring by chance). However, the use of correlational analysis has limited value since it is not unusual for high performance on one variable to correlate with high performance on another when the items tested are so similar in form. Further, it is only those who had reached a certain level of mastery on the NP variables who were predicted to do well on AUX, but restricting a data set in correlational analysis would obscure important relationships.

Overall NP and AUX Performance

As an alternative to this analysis the data were subjected to a series of t tests which allowed the L1 groups to be compared across proficiency levels.

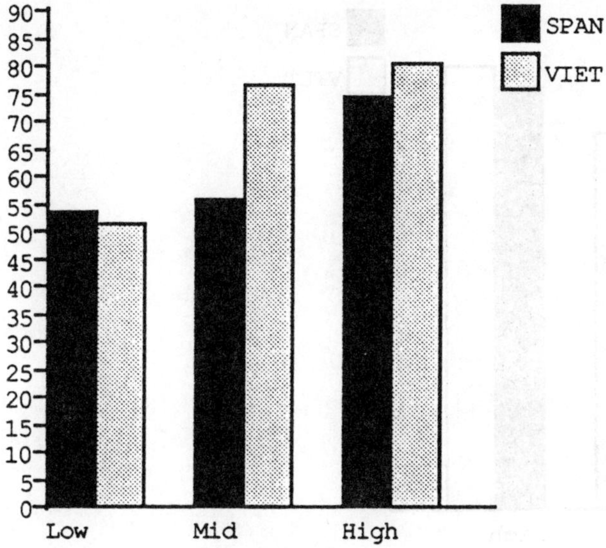

Figure 1. Performance on NP variables by L1 and proficiency level.

When Spanish and Vietnamese overall performance on NP and AUX variables was compared, the most striking finding was that Spanish speakers in the middle group (composed of 22 subjects, by far the largest group) scored almost as poorly as those in the lowest group, while the Vietnamese in that group on the average performed at about 75% correct. This result, shown in Figure 1, was unanticipated. Since both L1s license null subjects, by both transfer and developmental hypotheses the performance on this overall variable should be similar. This result also challenges the parameter-setting prediction, strongly suggesting that the knowledge that subjects are obligatory is not an early feature of English acquisition by adult Spanish speakers. (Numbers on the y axis are percentages.)

However, the groups performed similarly on the AUX variables, as in Figure 2, the cross-sectional data similar to a normal acquisition pattern. Although the developmental hypothesis predicted similar performance for the two groups on AUX, the transfer hypothesis predicted that Vietnamese speakers would have greater difficulty, thus score less well.

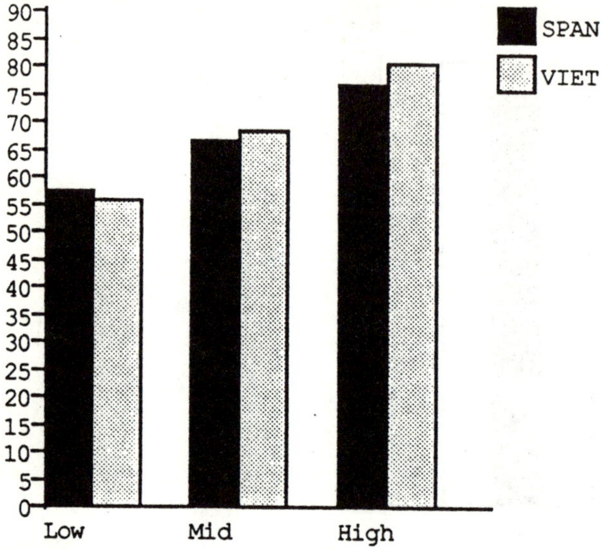

Figure 2. Performance on AUX variables by L1 and proficiency level.

When within L1 group comparisons made using the two main variables across the levels, the middle level Spanish speakers show less overall NP knowledge than AUX knowledge, challenging the second, or expletive trigger hypothesis. The Vietnamese, on the other hand demonstrate that at the middle level their NP knowledge exceeds AUX knowledge. Considering the very similar performance by both groups on the AUX variables, and the equal size increments between low and middle and between middle and high levels on those variables, the performance on the NP variables by middle level L1 groups is particularly interesting by contrast.

Orders of Difficulty

Although orders of difficulty of the different variables by all subjects can only suggest how higher level subjects performed, these data should indicate the presence of an expletive trigger for the Spanish speakers. However, aggregate data of the twelve individual variables show consistent higher levels of performance on AUX than on the NP variables. Figures 3 and 4 show order of difficulty of the for Spanish and Vietnamese speakers respectively. Figure 3 shows that the four AUX variables testing presence or absence of auxiliaries and position of auxiliaries with respect to *not* were easier than NP variables, particularly expletives. No cluster of either variable type was shown by the Vietnamese speakers, indicating that neither variable type was more difficult for this group. The list below is the key to the variable names used in the figures.

RFS	referential pronouns, singular
RFP	referential pronouns, plural
WIT	weather *it*
RIT	raising *it*
THS	there with singular
THP	*there* with plural
PABE	presence or absence of *be*
PAMO	presence or absence of modal
NOBE	position of *not* with *be*
NOMO	position of *not* with modal
VMBE	presence or absence of *be* with aspect marked
VMMO	presence or absence of modal with tensed verb

Individual Performance on Combined Variables

The final test of the second hypothesis was to see if for any subject the knowledge of expletives to a certain criterion preceded the reaching of the same criterion on AUX variables.[3] In order to accomplish that task, three combined variables were created representing each of the possible triggers: referential pronouns, expletive pronouns and auxiliaries. Only the four variables testing the presence or absence of AUX and the position of AUX with respect to *not* were used for this final test, since the verb-marking variables were considered to be logical extensions of the definition "AUX knowledge," but not inherent in the original Hyams characterization. For purposes of this analysis only the data of subjects who had reached a criterion on any two out of three of the combined variables were examined, since evidence for a triggering stage requires that two kinds of knowledge be mastered, the trigger, and the triggered knowledge. Those who had achieved criterion on one or no variables were considered not to have reached the parameter-setting stage (or lacked the proficiency to respond to the test items.) Those who achieved criterion on all three variables were assumed to be beyond

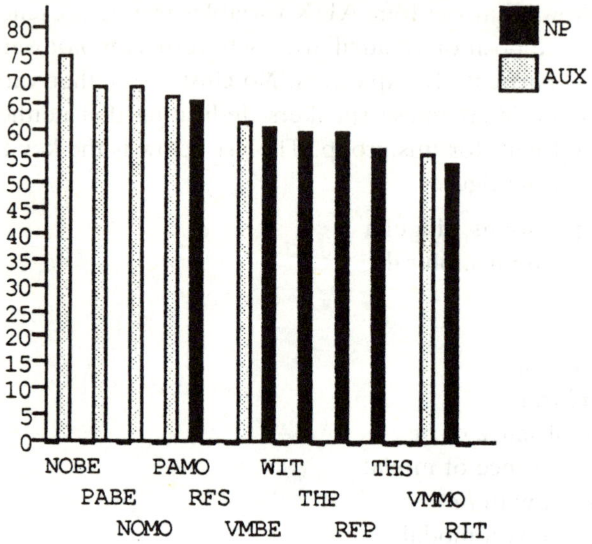

Figure 3. Order of difficulty of all variables for Spanish group.

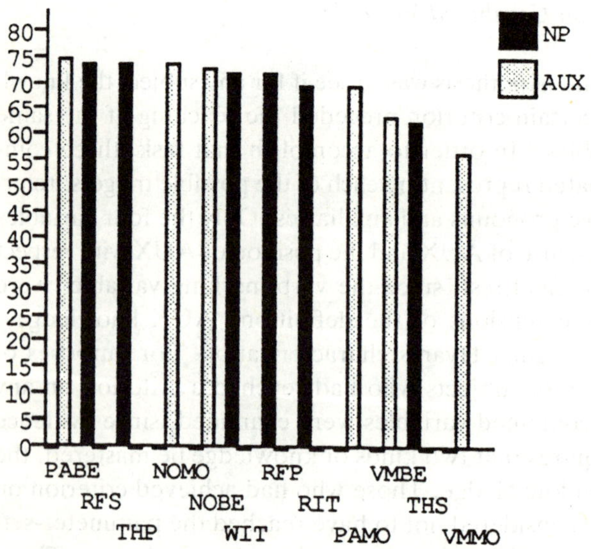

Figure 4. Order of difficulty of all variables for Vietnamese group.

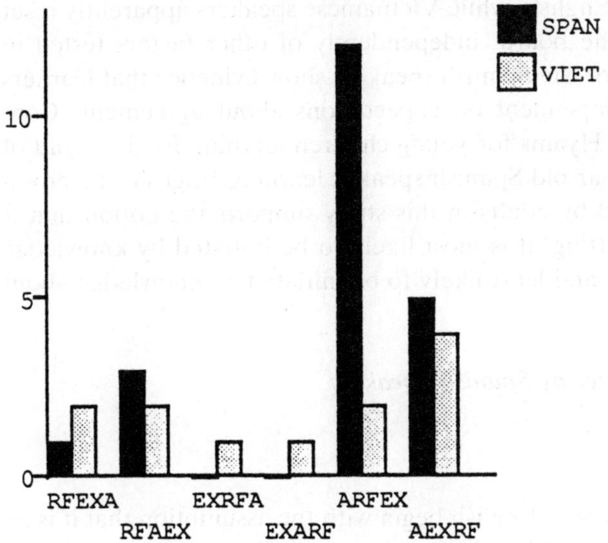

Figure 5. Individual mastery orders for both L1 groups

the triggering stage. When the individual mastery orders were examined, a preference for an AUX first order was found for the Spanish speakers. *Not one* of the subjects who were in the triggering stage reached criterion on expletives first, the final piece of evidence against the second hypothesis. On the other hand, the Vietnamese subjects showed no particular mastery order, and no constraints on orders, as shown in Figure 5. Variable names for the figure are as follows: RF - referential pronouns, EX - expletive, and A - auxiliaries. X axis labels show possible orders of the three variables. Numbers on the y axis are numbers of subjects. Gaps in EXRFA and EXARF mean that no Spanish speakers displayed the order.

Discussion

In this section the results of this study are discussed in terms of plausible levels of understanding held by both Spanish and Vietnamese speakers for the resetting of the null subject parameter. Spanish speakers appear to proceed through three stages to reset the null subject parameter in accordance with the facts of English, while Vietnamese speakers apparently reset the parameter across the board, independently of other factors tested in this study. The stages for the Spanish speakers show evidence that learners construct hypotheses dependent on expectations about agreement. Contrary to the findings of Hyams for young children learning English, and of Hilles for her twelve year-old Spanish speaker learning English, the cross-sectional data produced by adults in this study supports the notion that if there is parameter-resetting, it is most likely to be initiated by knowledge about AUX and AGR, and least likely to be initiated by knowledge about the status of subjects.

Resetting of the Parameter by Spanish Speakers

The First Stage

Spanish-speaking learners of English begin with the assumption that it is an agreement language. Several kinds of evidence support this hypothesis and the consequent belief that English allows null subjects. First, Spanish speakers encountering English hear different endings on verb stems — *-ing*, *-s*, and *-ed* as well as irregular past and participial forms which are similar enough to their infinitival counterparts to be recognized. But at first they do not know whether these are tense or agreement endings. The copula *be* has an incomplete agreement paradigm, but it is so common that it must provide learners with strong evidence for agreement. It is not obvious that Spanish speakers immediately recognize that *be* with *-ing* affixed to the verb is the same thing as estar + verb + -ando and its allomorphs. Many speakers accept the progressive aspect stem without *be*, and even more accept a form of *be* plus verb without *-ing*. The fact that subjects performed better on *not* variables than on those testing presence or absence of *be* and modals suggests that when Spanish speakers still accept null referential subjects, they apparently recognize that AUX is not in VP. This occurs even before they know the possible contents of AUX, contrary to the evidence from English L1 acquisition. Learners in late Stage 1 have begun to reset the parameter.

The Second Stage

The second stage for the Spanish speakers is characterized by the correct knowledge that English AGR is too impoverished to identify null referential subjects, since only the third person singular suffix marks agreement in present tense. Thus, they have learned that the identification condition on null subjects does not hold for English. Evidence for this knowledge is that Spanish speakers as a whole mastered the singular referential pronoun variable to the same level as the variable testing presence or absence of a modal. (This variable may actually have tested sensitivity to the presence or absence of the third person singular, for each of the incorrect sentences could be made correct with the addition of *-s* to the verb.) However, recognition that AGR cannot identify subjects in English does not suffice to induce full parameter resetting, for the learner in this stage still has not learned that expletive deletion is not licensed. Learners in late Stage 2 are near the end of the parameter-resetting stage.

The Third Stage

When Spanish speakers have reset the parameter, they have internalized the fact that neither identification nor licensing conditions are met for the deletion of subject pronominals in English. Evidence that expletives cannot provide the trigger for AUX restructuring should be found in the performance of the high group. But the performance of the most proficient Spanish speakers shows that while thematic subjects reach a level of about 80%, performance on expletives ranges from 65-75%, the lowest variable being raising *it*. This indicates a lag in the development of knowledge that null expletives are not licensed in English, only a few of the subjects tested in this study having reset the parameter completely. This apparent lag may therefore point to a constraint on the resetting of this parameter: expletives cannot provide the triggering data, if "trigger" refers to earliest mastered knowledge, because Spanish learners must first discover that English is not an AGR language. However, that information does not automatically confer knowledge about expletives. Since referential subjects cannot be identified in English, they cannot be null. And since expletives lack an identification requirement, the learners still have not learned the very abstract concept that null non-thematic subjects are not licensed in English.[4] Only when Spanish speakers internalize the positive evidence that all tensed clauses contain either referential or expletive subjects, and perhaps some negative evidence that null subjects are disallowed, can they be said to have reset the parameter, thus restructuring the early grammar.

Resetting of the Parameter by Vietnamese Speakers

The Vietnamese data differ from the Spanish in that both referential and expletive subjects were mastered to about the same level by subjects at the middle level of proficiency. Also, the Vietnamese performed similarly on the two NP types. Thus, inherent complexity of expletives alone can not explain the difference between the referential and expletive performance by the Spanish speakers at the highest proficiency level. One possible reason for the strong performance of the Vietnamese speakers in the middle group on all the NP variables is that the Vietnamese speakers, without a strong identification requirement in L1, realize early that English requires identification of subjects. In the theoretical section two alternative possibilities were presented for the Vietnamese speakers, 1) considerable difficulty learning to supply NPs in their appropriate environments, or 2) early learning from positive evidence of expletives. Consistent with written data collected from Vietnamese-speaking learners of English (see Platt 1989), the subjects in this study appeared to know that English tensed clauses require subjects. However, just because Vietnamese learners of English know that a subject is required does not mean that they always fill the position correctly. Sentence (16) below shows a locative filling the subject role, while (17) shows overgeneralizing of contexts for subjects.

(16) In Vietnam have a lot of people die.

(17) The boy get on the bus and he go to school and he take his lunch.

If the subjects had had to judge such sentences, they may have experienced greater difficulty. Further, their difficulty with singular *there* shows that while they may have had a slot for subjects in tensed clauses, they had not worked out the differences between the semantic properties of the Vietnamese *có* and the English existential *there*. This explanation relies to some extent on subjects' ability to distinguish between tensed and untensed clauses in English, as pointed out earlier, so they probably do not use it in their early hypotheses about how English works. Since the instrument did not test presence or absence of subjects in untensed clauses, it is not possible to state with confidence whether the participants in this study knew that the sentences required subjects because of the tensing of the clause, or because of some other factor not tested.[5] The specification of the parameter which accounts for null subjects in Vietnamese requires further analysis of the features of that language which are directly related to NP deletion. Until that analysis has been made, an explanation of the early resetting of the parameter consistent with English must remain speculative.[6]

Alternative Explanations

Although neither surface level transfer nor developmental hypotheses provide global explanations of this study's findings, both explain some of them. The strongest evidence for transfer is the expletive performance by both L1 groups. Differences between singular and plural *there* demonstrated by Vietnamese speakers, and between weather and raising *it* shown by the Spanish speakers, while not statistically significant, nonetheless suggest that the semantic properties of expletives are as important as their grammatical properties in acquisition. Evidence consistent with a developmental hypothesis is found in the very similar performance by both groups on the AUX variables. Also, assuming the generalizability of cross-sectional data to the course of development for an individual, additional evidence for this view lies in the fact that parameter-resetting is not an instantaneous occurrence, but a gradual process. The fact that stages have been posited reflects the developmental view.

The parameter-setting hypothesis goes beyond either surface transfer or developmental hypotheses, attempting explanation of phenomena theoretically related by syntactic principles, in this case the occurrence of null subjects in two different types of null subject languages, one having AGR, the other not. The results produced by many of the Vietnamese subjects are consistent with the child English acquisition data cited by Hyams in her work. The composite scores of the Vietnamese-speaking subjects on NP and AUX increased incrementally across proficiency levels. Two reasons possibly explain the similarity in NP and AUX performance for the Vietnamese. First, item types were similar in all parts of the task. Subjects were required to look and listen for bound or free morphemes that were missing and for morphemes in the wrong order. Second, as revealed by the fact that children demonstrate roughly simultaneous acquisition of unstressed referential pronouns, expletives and common auxiliaries, these features may be perceived as inherently equally abstract or complex. In addition to their being syntactic phenomena, the features tested also contain semantic content, and the properties of the semantic notions expressed by them must be acknowledged in a full explanation of their acquisition. The fact that the relationship predicted by the Hyams hypothesis was demonstrated by the Vietnamese to a greater extent than by the Spanish speakers points to a possible inhibitory rather than a facilitative relationship between NP and AUX knowledge for the latter.

The relationship of the the constructs NP and AUX knowledge was found for the Spanish speakers in the orders of difficulty of the AUX and NP variables, the combined AUX variable being performed better than any of the NP variables. No evidence for an expletive trigger was found since no Spanish speakers in the triggering stage reached criterion on expletives before doing so on either referential pronouns or auxiliaries.[7] Alternatively, the data support the notion of a constraint on the acquisition of the overt expletive until certain other knowledge has been attained, namely that relating to agreement and to the identification of referential pronouns. Unlike child learners of English, who never have evidence that English is an agreement language, Spanish speakers must first learn that English is not such a language. Only after finding out that null pronominals are not identified and expletives are not licensed do Spanish speakers acquire full knowledge of the English obligatory subject. There being no linkage of empty elements and auxiliaries in Vietnamese, and there being no agreement at all, Vietnamese speakers construct hypotheses about NP and AUX independently, and apparently at about the same time.

Conclusions

Because the differential NP performance by the two L1 groups cannot be accounted for by either developmental nor surface transfer theories, the results of this study require an explanation of a different sort. The parameter-setting framework provides a plausible theoretical structure within which such explanation is possible. Analyses within this framework have already suggested to both first and second language acquisition researchers that the the abstract underlying relationship of empty categories to other properties of null subject languages might have some psychological reality which can be identified by various elicitation or judgment tasks. This study tested four hypotheses related to the Hyams (1986) claim for child learners.

While its findings strongly challenge the postulated directionality of acquisition by the Spanish speakers of the parametrically-related features, they nonetheless support the notion of a relationship between them. It has been argued here that the relationship is inhibitory. Acquisition of overt expletives cannot occur until the proper conditions for first identification, then licensing, are found lacking in English, these conditions being linked to the agreement features of languages of this type. The data point to the possibility that these two conditions are different for Spanish speakers, as evidenced by their poor overall performance on expletive items as compared with referential pronoun items.

Performance by the Vietnamese speakers suggests that no inhibitory relationships occur between the two features, since they scored similarly on both NP and AUX variables. It further points to the possibility that the lack of a strong identification requirement in Vietnamese does not carry over to learners' hypotheses about English, for items testing presence or absence of both referential and expletive pronouns were performed similarly by this L1 group at the middle level, and significantly better than their Spanish counterparts. These puzzling findings are not altogether satisfactorily explained, but advances in syntactic analysis of Southeast Asian languages should assist SLA researchers in finding testable hypotheses for speakers of these languages. A more adequate explanation is required for why unrelated languages, both with null subjects, have different underlying representations of these elements, manifested in interesting ways in SLA. To date no hypothesis within the principles and parameters framework can account for the differences. Research of this type clearly points to the need for an eventual reconciliation of language-specific and general cognitive models. While syntactic theory attempts to explain abstract relationships among properties of languages, more elaborated theories of cognitive complexity are needed to explain under what conditions these relationships are most likely to be revealed.

Notes

1. Alternatively, by the Morphological Uniformity Principle (Jaeggli and Hyams 1987), licensing is accomplished by the uniformity of zero morphological marking across the board.
2. Cole (1987) argues convincingly for the occurrence of *pro* in object position in Thai, Korean and some varieties of Quechua.

3. "Criterion," about 72%, represents performance significantly above the limits of chance, though not mastery as a score of 90% or better would represent. The lower score was selected as a criterion in order to identify enough Spanish-speaking subjects to justify the use of parametric statistical procedures.

4. The claim that licensing of null expletives as a class follows from rich agreement is a problem in the Hyams (1986) hypothesis. In languages like Spanish and Italian AGR identifies null referential subjects, but does not license null expletives, for which there is no identification requirement. The Morphological Uniformity Principle (Jaeggli and Hyams 1987) distinguishes between these two conditions, accounting for null expletive licensing by morphological uniformity.

5. It is common in Vietnamese for sentences to begin with locative or temporal adverbials, the latter being used to establish the temporal frame of the discourse. One of the reasons for designing the test items with either prepositional phrases or subordinate clauses in initial position was to avoid the possibility that Vietnamese speakers would reject items for discourse-pragmatic rather than syntactic reasons.

6. Namtip Pingkarawat's (1989) dissertation on null NPs and control in Thai provides much of this needed information.

7. More recent work of both Hilles (1991) and Hyams (Hyams 1987; Jaeggli and Hyams 1987) also refutes the expletive trigger notion.

References

Adams, Marianne. 1987. "From Old French to the Theory of Pro-drop". *Natural Language and Linguistic Theory* 5.1-32.

Aoun, Joseph, and Dominique Sportiche. 1983. "On the Formal Theory of Government". *The Linguistic Review* 2.211-236.

Bellugi, U. 1967. *The Acquisition of Negation*. Unpublished doctoral dissertation, Harvard University, Boston, Mass.

Bloom, L. 1970. *Language Development: Form and Function in Emerging Grammars*. Cambridge, MA: MIT Press

Brown, Roger, and C. Fraser. 1964. "The Acquisition of Syntax". *The Acquisition of Language* ed. by Ursula Bellugi and Roger Brown, 43-100. Chicago: University of Chicago Press.

Chomsky, Noam. 1965. *Aspects of the Theory of Syntax*. Cambridge, MA: MIT Press.

Chomsky, Noam. 1981. *Lectures on Government and Binding*. Dordrecht: Foris.

Chomsky, Noam. 1986. *Knowledge of Language*. New York: Praeger.

Cole, Peter. 1987. "Null Objects in UG". *Linguistic Inquiry* 18.97-612.

Cook, V.J. 1985. "Universal Grammar and Second Language Learning". *Applied Linguistics* 6.2-18.

Flynn, Suzanne, and Wayne O'Neil. 1988. "Introduction". *Linguistic Theory in Second Language Acquisition* ed. by Suzanne Flynn and Wayne O'Neil, 1-24. Dordrecht: Kluwer Academic Publishers.

Guilfoyle, Eithne. 1984. "The Acquisition of Tense and the Emergence of Lexical Subjects". *McGill University Working Papers in Linguistics* 20-30.

Hermon, Gabriella and James Yoon. 1989. "The Licensing and Identification of pro and the Typology of AGR". Chicago: Chicago Linguistic Society.

Hilles, Sharon. 1986. "Interlanguage and the Pro-drop Parameter". *Second Language Research* 2.33-52.

Hilles, Sharon. 1991. "Access to Universal Grammar in Second Language Acquisition". *Point Counterpoint: Universal Grammar in Second Language* ed. by Lynn Eubank. Amsterdam: John Benjamins.

Hoa, Dinh Nguyen. 1966. *Speak Vietnamese*. Rutland, Vt.: Charles E. Tuttle Co.

Huang, C.T. James. 1984a. "On the Distribution and Reference of Empty Categories". *Linguistic Inquiry* 15.531-574.

Huang, C.T. James. 1984b. "On the Typology of Zero Anaphora". *Language Research* 20.85-105.

Huang, C. T. James. 1989. "Pro-drop in Chinese: A Generalized Control Approach".

Hyams, Nina. M. 1986. *Language Acquisition and the Theory of Parameters*. Dordrecht: D. Reidel Publishing Company.

Hyams, Nina. M. 1987. "The Setting of the Null Subject Parameter". Paper presented at the Boston University Conference on Child Language Development, Boston, Mass.

Jaeggli, Oswaldo. and Nina Hyams. 1987. "Morphological Uniformity and the Setting of the Null Subject Parameter". Unpublished manuscript, University of Southern California, Los Angeles.

Johnson, Jackie. 1988. *Critical period effects on universal properties of language: The status of subjacency in the acquisition of a second language*. Unpublished doctoral dissertation, University of Illinois, Urbana-Champaign.

Johnson, Jackie. and Elissa Newport. 1989. "Critical Period Effects in Second Language Learning: The Influence of Maturational State on the Acquisition of English as a Second Language". *Cognitive Psychology* 21.60-99.

Lado, Robert. 1983. Excerpts from "Linguistics across cultures." *Second Language Learning: Contrastive Analysis, Error Analysis and Related Aspects* ed. by Betty W. Robinette and Jacquelyn Schachter, 21-32. Ann Arbor: University of Michigan Press.

Lebeaux, David. 1987. "Comments on Hyams". Roeper and Williams 1987.23-39.

Lehman, F. K.1988. "Problems in the Syntax of Verb Concatenation in Burmese". Draft paper for the Nineteenth Annual International Conference on Sino-Tibetan Languages and Linguistics.

Lehman, F.K. and Namtip Pingkarawat. 1985. "Missing Nominals, Non-specificity and Related Matters, with Special Reference to Thai and Burmese". *Studies in the Linguistics Sciences* 15.101-121.

Major, Diane. 1974. *The Acquisition of Modal Auxiliaries in the Language of Children*. The Hague: Mouton.

Newport, Elissa, and Ted Supalla. Forthcoming. "A Critical Period Effect in the Acquisition of a Primary Language". To appear in *Science*.

Phinney, Marianne. 1987. "The Pro-drop Parameter in Second Language Acquisition". Roeper and Williams 1987.221-238.

Pingkarawat, Namtip. 1989. *Empty noun phrases and the theory of control with special reference to Thai*. Unpublished doctoral dissertation, University of Illinois, Urbana-Champaign.

Platt, Elizabeth J. 1989. "Testing the Null Subject Parameter in Adult SLA: A Study of Vietnamese and Spanish Speakers Learning English. Unpublished doctoral dissertation, University of Illinois, Urbana-Champaign.

Roeper, Thomas and Edwin Williams. 1987. *Parameter Setting*. Dordrrecht: D. Reidel.

Rizzi, Luigi. 1982. "Negation, Wh-movement and the Null Subject Parameter". *Issues in Italian Syntax* ed. by Luigi Rizzi, 117-184. Dordrecht: Foris.

Rizzi, Luigi. 1986. "Null Objects in Italian". *Linguistic Inquiry* 17.501-557.

Suñer, Margaret. 1982. "On Null Subjects". *Linguistic Analysis* 9.55-78.

White, Lydia. 1984. "Universal Grammar as a Source of Explanation in Second-language Acquisition" *Current Approaches to Second Language Acquisition* ed. by B. Wheatley, A. Hastings, F. Eckman, L. Bell, G. Krukar and R. Rutkowski, 43-68. Bloomington, IN: Indiana University Linguistics club.

White, Lydia. 1985. "The Pro-drop Parameter in Adult Second Language Acquisition". *Language Learning* 35.47-62.

Linguistics and Speech-Language Pathology

Individual Differences in Phonological Disorders and Implications for a Theory of Acquisition

Daniel A. Dinnsen and Steven B. Chin
Department of Linguistics, Indiana University

Linguists are primarily concerned with constructing and testing theories of natural language. These theories are expected to account for the full range of variation across the world's languages. In this regard, linguists are always looking for new and exotic languages or language phenomena to test the efficacy of some particular theoretical construct, relationship, process, or mechanism. The standard domain of linguistic investigation seems, however, to be limited to fully developed primary languages. This means that the interlanguage systems of second language learners and the disordered systems associated with speech-language pathologies are not considered 'natural languages' in the same sense and thus have not served as a crucial source of linguistic variation relevant to linguistic theory.

It is also generally acknowledged that any theory that can account for the process of language acquisition is to be preferred. Facts about first language acquisition are thus of obvious and undisputed relevance. Again, however, facts about second language acquisition and acquisition associated with speech-language pathologies are viewed differently and have not enjoyed central relevance to the acquisition process. To the extent that second language acquisition is like first language acquisition, it too can serve as an appropriate testing ground for linguistic theory. The interlanguage systems of second language learners are also certainly describable within the limits of current linguistic theory (e.g., Adjemian, 1976; Eckman, 1987; Selinker, 1972) and as such constitute another legitimate domain for the examination of linguistic systems that may present phenomena or structures relevant to theoretical concerns.

Linguistic systems associated with speech or language pathologies have also been described within various theoretical frameworks (e.g., Crystal

1980; Ingram 1976); however, their relevance to theory or the acquisition process has been more tenuous. More specifically, facts about disordered systems have not figured into any arguments for a particular conception of language or for any theoretical construct. The assumption seems to have been that disordered systems are somehow deviant in nature and thus unlike any other language system. Speech-language pathologists have fostered this view by their continued reliance on behavioral models of language and, in at least the case of misarticulation or phonological disorders, their assumption that errors are the result of motor deficiencies or simplification processes that are themselves based largely in motor or perceptual limitations. Little about the disorder has to do with the nature of language itself. It is thus not surprising that there are so few linguistic descriptions of disordered systems and that speech pathologists rely so little on linguistic principles in the planning and execution of remediation programs. It is no less surprising that linguists have not relied on disordered systems in the evaluation and construction of theories about language. After all, there are few descriptions available to provide any real information about the nature of disordered systems, and the population of speakers is accessible only through clinically certified investigators.

This conception of disorders by both linguists and speech-language pathologists is unfortunate, since it embodies such an important but possibly unnecessary or incorrect assumption about the nature of disorders. If no a priori assumption were made about disorders, descriptions of disordered systems could be developed on empirical grounds and compared with normal first acquired systems at any and all stages of development. To the extent that such comparisons failed to identify substantive or functional differences, disordered systems would constitute a legitimate domain for the construction and evaluation of liguistic theory.

The purpose of this paper is twofold: (1) to illustrate the applicability of linguistic theory to the description of disordered phonological systems when no a priori assumption is made about the nature of disorders, and (2) to consider the implications of those descriptions for linguistic theory and the process of acquisition. To this end, a series of collaborative studies will be summarized.

The work of David Ingram (1976, 1981) has probably had the most profound impact on descriptions of phonological disorders. His work has revealed that children's errors can be described by phonological rules (or processes) that express a systematic relationship with the target system. For example, a child who systematically substitutes [t] for [s] would be claimed to have a rule of 'stopping' in his phonology. The emphasis of most current work has thus focused on error patterns and the rules accounting for those patterns. The general assumption has been that the rules operate on correct underlying representations. In the case of a 'stopping' process, it would be assumed that the child knows at the underlying level of representation that words are represented with /s/ even if no words are ever realized phonetically with [s]. The nature of underlying representations in any phonological system is a fundamental characteristic of that system. It is thus important to the characterization of disordered systems to know, based on empirical considerations, whether the disorder relates to differences in the phonological rules or the underlying representations or both. In one of our earliest studies (Weismer, Dinnsen, and Elbert 1981), the a priori assumption that underlying representations are correct for this population was challenged and argued to be neither necessary nor sufficient. In that study, the phonological and phonetic properties of a single error pattern, final consonant omission, common to the three children in that study were examined. The problem was to determine whether there were empirical grounds for claims about the characterization of the error pattern and if those claims were the same across subjects exhibiting the same error pattern. Morphophonemically relevant data for two of the subjects are presented in (1) (data from Weismer, et al., 1981, and Dinnsen and Maxwell 1981).

(1) Final Consonant Omission (Weismer, Dinnsen, and Elbert 1981; Dinnsen and Maxwell 1981)

Subject A (Age 7;2)		Subject C (Age 3;6)	
[kæ:] 'cab'	[kæbi] 'cabby'		
[ka] 'cop'	[kapoʊ] 'copper'		
[kι:] 'kid'	[kidoʊ] 'kidder'	[dæ] 'dad'	[dæi] 'daddy'
[pæ] 'pat'	[pæti] 'patty'	[i] 'eat'	[iin] 'eating'
[dɔ:] 'dog'	[dɔgi] 'doggie'	[da] 'dog'	[dai] 'doggie'
[dʌ] 'duck'	[dʌki] 'ducky'		

As can be seen, both subjects omitted final obstruents. However, a crucial fact differentiated the two. Subject A exhibited an alternation between obstruents medially and null word-finally. Subject C, on the other hand, exhibited no alternation and failed to realize obstruents in any word-internal post-vocalic context. Based on strictly empirical considerations (the same considerations that would be employed to motivate claims about any primary language), it was maintained that Subject A correctly represented morphemes with post-vocalic obstruents at the underlying level but deleted them by a phonological rule in a specific, well-defined context, namely word-final position. The facts for Subject C failed to support any claim of correct underlying representations or a rule deleting obstruents. The absence of post-vocalic obstruents was attributed to a positional constraint that excluded post-vocalic obstruents at all levels of representation. Subject C thus represented these morphemes incorrectly at the underlying level. The correctness of these analyses was further supported by an instrumental and experimental investigation of vowel length before omitted final obstruents for these same subjects. It was found that Subject A maintained a systematic vowel length difference before omitted voiced and voiceless obstruents such that vowels were relatively long before omitted voiced obstruents and relatively short before omitted voiceless obstruents. The facts about the alternation and vowel length converge to show that Subject A had underlying knowledge about the omitted obstruents. Subject C failed to maintain any such vowel length differences and thus failed again to evidence any knowledge of the omitted obstruents. These results demonstrated that a given error pattern can derive from either correct or incorrect underlying representations. Moreover, claims about the nature of the underlying representations were shown to be motivated on empirical grounds and thus required no a priori assumptions.

Admitting a distinction between correct and incorrect underlying representations in the characterization of error patterns predicts a broad range of linguistic variation both within and across error patterns and within and across subjects. Thus, as in the case above, a given error pattern across different subjects can derive from different underlying representations (correct or incorrect). Also, different error patterns within and across subjects can derive from the same underlying representations (either all correct or all incorrect) by the application (or nonapplication) of phonological rules (e.g., Gierut, Elbert, and Dinnsen 1987). The range of variation is further augmented if one considers that it is equally possible that a child's correct productions could in principle also derive from either correct or incorrect underlying representations. It is an empirical issue whether such variation actually occurs. If it does, linguistic theory will have motivated a refocusing away from error patterns alone to the child's total system, which includes both correct and incorrect productions. The clinical significance of this new focus would be that linguistic problems may underlie even correct productions.

In a recent study (Dinnsen and Chin 1988), the phonological systems of 40 young children with moderate to severe functional (nonorganic) speech disorders were examined. Subjects exhibited a variety of error patterns along with a complementary set of correct productions. In order to account for the production facts of those systems, it was necessary to appeal to correct and incorrect underlying representations and to the application and nonapplication of various phonological rules. These theoretical constructs combined in all logically possible ways to yield the full range of variation predicted. The results are summarized in (2) and (3) below.

Given the possibilities of either correct or incorrect phonetic representations and either correct or incorrect underlying representations, we arrive at the four logical possibilities for rule-governed phenomena given in (2).

(2) Rule-Governed Phenomena

a. Correct Underlying Representation - Correct Phonetic Representation (Subject 13)
[p^{h}ʊ] 'push' [bæk] 'back'
[t^{h}ʌ:] 'tub' [daʊ] 'door'
[k^{h}ʌp] 'cup' [gʌm] 'gum'
[-son, -cont, -voice] → [+asp] / # ____

b. Correct Underlying Representation - Incorrect Phonetic Representation (Subject 22)
[bʌs] / [bʌʃιn] 'brush/brushing'
[wιts] / [wιtʃi] 'witch/witchie'
[k^{h}eιdz] / [k^{h}eιdʒi] 'cage/cagey'
but
[bʌs] / [bʌsi] 'bus/bussy'
[+cor] → [+ant] / ____ #

c. Incorrect Underlying Representation - Correct Phonetic Representation (Subject 35)
[p^{h}iʃi] / [p^{h}itʃ] 'peachy/peach'
[wιʃi] / [wιtʃ] 'witchie/witch'
[k^{h}æʃiŋ] / [k^{h}ætʃ] 'catching/catch'
[wɑʃi] / [wɑtʃ] 'watchie/watch'
but also
[bʌʃən] / [b^{w}ʌtʃ] 'brushing/brush'
[fιʃιŋ] / [fιtʃ] 'fishing/fish'
[−ant] → [−cont] / ____ #

d. Incorrect Underlying Representation - Incorrect Phonetic Representation (Subject 23)
[wɛdi] / [wɛ] 'webby/web'
[bɛgi] / [bɛ] 'beddy/bed'
[pʰɩdi] / [pʰɩ] 'piggy/pig'
but
[tʰʌti] / [tʰʌt] 'cutting/cut'
[pʰʌpi] / [pʰʌp] 'cuppy/cup'
$[+\text{cons}, +\text{voice}] \rightarrow \emptyset$ / ____ #

Number (2a) presents an example of (at least partially) correct productions derived from correct underlying representations. In this particular case, the child evidenced a voice contrast word-initially and correctly aspirated the voiceless stops by means of the English allophonic rule, resulting in certain aspects of the words being produced correctly. Although this aspect of the child's phonology corresponded with the target system, this same child evidenced multiple errors on other aspects of his speech. At least as regards the underlying and phonetic representation of voiced and voiceless obstruents in word-initial position, the child's system corresponds perfectly with English and would not represent a clinical concern.

Number (2b) is an example of incorrect productions derived from correct underlying representations by means of a phonological rule that fronts palatoalveolar fricatives and affricates word finally. The claim in this case is that the child has target-appropriate knowledge of palatoalveolar fricatives and affricates in all word positions; the error is accounted for by a non-English phonological rule. Clinically, then, the elimination of the rule should result in correct productions.

Example (2c) is perhaps the most interesting and insidious possibility. In this case, the child evidences some correct productions for the wrong reasons.[1] In this particular example, affricates are produced correctly in word-final position in some words but are derived from incorrect underlying representations involving fricatives. For this child, affricates and fricatives contrast in word-initial position but do not contrast post-vocalically. There is moreover an alternation such that fricatives occur word-medially and affricates occur word-finally. A non-English phonological rule of word-final affrication accounts for the alternation. Even if the opposite directionality (deaffrication or spirantization word medially) were assumed, some correct productions would derive from incorrect underlying representations in word-medial position. The result is that English words with final affricates or medial fricatives appear to be produced correctly. On the other hand, English words with final fricatives or medial affricates are produced incorrectly. Other cases of this sort have been reported in the literature but have not been recognized as instances of correct productions for the wrong reasons (e.g., Camarata and Gandour 1984; Gierut 1986; Williams and Dinnsen 1987). Clinically, these are interesting cases because they might have gone unnoticed if morphophonemically related forms had not been elicited and because they require the restructuring of underlying representations and the elimination of a non-English rule in order to bring that aspect of the system into conformity with the target system.

Example (2d) presents a case of incorrect productions derived from incorrect underlying representations by a non-English rule deleting voiced obstruents word-finally. The alternation reveals the incorrectness of the underlying representations; that is, when a morpheme-final voiced obstruent is realized medially, it is the wrong obstruent. The alternate realization of the morpheme without a final voiced obstruent is also incorrect, but its incorrectness is due to a non-English rule deleting voiced obstruents word-finally. In such cases, the production facts are completely in error, because both the underlying representations and the rule are wrong.

The listing in (3) presents the same range of possibilities, except that no rule mediates between the levels of representation.

(3) Non-Rule-Governed Phenomena

a. Correct Underlying Representation - Correct Phonetic Representation (Subject 16)
[bɛd] / [bɛdi] ‘bed/beddy’
[wɛb] / [wɛbi] ‘web/webby’
[mun] / [muni] ‘moon/moonie’
[wɩm] / [wɩmɩn] ‘swim/swimming’

b. Correct Underlying Representation - Incorrect Phonetic Representation (Subject 29)
[peɩdʒi] ‘pagey’
[puˀtiŋ] ‘pushing’
and
[bɛɾi] ‘beddy’
[bʊki] ‘booky’

c. Incorrect Underlying Representation - Correct Phonetic Representation (Subject 21)
[dɪps] 'chips'
[g̥ɑts] 'cats'
[g̥eɪks] 'cakes'
but also
[taʊs] 'toes'
[g̥aʊms] 'combs'
[g̥aɪvs] 'caves'
[waʊz] 'rose'
[tiz] 'cheese'

d. Incorrect Underlying Representation - Incorrect Phonetic Representation (Subject 27)
[t^{h}if] / [t^{h}ifi] 'teeth/teethy'
[bæf] / [bæfi] 'bath/bathy'
[maʊf] / [maʊfi] 'mouth/mouthy'

Example (3a) illustrates a portion of a speech disordered system that is completely target-appropriate. That is, at least nasals and voiced stops are realized correctly in all contexts and do not alternate. These sounds thus represent no problem for any aspect of this subject's phonology. There were, of course, many other aspects of this subject's phonology that were in error.

Example (3b) presents a case of incorrect productions that derive from correct underlying representations where the English rule of aspiration should have applied but did not. In this particular case, the child correctly internalized the distinction between voiced and voiceless obstruents but failed to internalize the allophonic law of English pronunciation that aspirates voiceless stops word-initially. Such cases are clinically interesting because the child needs only to learn the English rule of aspiration. Typically, however, conventional treatment focuses on teaching phonemic contrasts rather than rules, and it remains unclear how allophonic rules of this sort would be taught.

Example (3c) presents another interesting case of correct productions for the wrong reasons. In this example, the plural is correctly realized in certain words but for very different reasons than in English. It is generally assumed for English that the plural morpheme is represented underlyingly as /z/, and that a rule of progressive devoicing accounts for the alternation (e.g., Shibatani 1972). In the present case, however, the plural does not alternate. It is always realized as [s] and thus would be represented as /s/ underlyingly. It should be noted moreover that this child does allow [z] word-finally but not in association with the plural morpheme. This child has thus internalized a phonemic distinction between /s/ and /z/ but not correctly in all morphemes. The correct realization of the plural for this child derives from an incorrect underlying representation with no intervening rule. This child needs to learn the correct underlying representation of the plural morpheme and the English rule of progressive devoicing if this aspect of his phonology is to be brought into conformity with English. Given the fundamental differences between allophonic and neutralizing rules (Houlihan and Iverson 1979), learning the progressive devoicing rule (neutralizing) may be more or less difficult than learning the aspiration rule (allophonic) relevant to the error in (3b). We might in addition expect that the task of teaching such different types of rules would also be different.

Number (3d) contains an example of incorrect productions resulting from incorrect underlying representations. These words were produced incorrectly and without alternation. [θ] did not occur anywhere in this child's phonetic inventory. This child's underlying and phonetic representations were thus presumed to be identical and of course incorrect. The learning task that confronts this child is different from that presented in (3c). Here the child must only restructure his underlying representations to include [θ]. In the case of (3c), the child must restructure the underlying representation of the plural morpheme and add the rule of progressive devoicing.

These examples illustrate the interaction of linguistic theory and speech pathology. First, phonological theory reveals speech disordered systems to be highly differentiated as a result of appeal to very basic linguistic constructs, namely the nature of a child's underlying representations and the application or nonapplication of a phonological rule. These disordered systems in turn represent learnable varieties of English or are at least learned systems that are related to English as described above. As such, they constitute a rich source of information about language variation and acquisition. The correctness of the phonological descriptions and their clinical relevance have been supported by studies that have examined individual differences in learning patterns. Dinnsen and Elbert (1984) and Gierut et al. (1987) have found through experimental treatment studies that children's learning patterns correspond with differential claims of phonological knowledge such that greater levels of performance are achieved on errored aspects of the phonology involving correct underlying representations. Important aspects of these claims remain to be experimentally tested. More specifically, the relative ease or difficulty of overcoming errors associated with rules versus no rule is unknown. It is likewise unknown whether correct productions derived from incorrect underlying representations present an especially difficult problem to reconcile due to the nontransparent relationship between the two systems.

Let us now turn our attention to variation in a more superficial aspect of disordered systems, namely the nature of phonetic inventories. In a recent study Dinnsen, Chin, Elbert, and Powell (1990) examined the pretreatment phonetic inventories of 34 functionally misarticulating children aged 3 years 4 months to 6 years 8 months. Considerable variation was observed across the inventories in terms of the number and type of sounds that occurred. In addition, there was no correlation between subjects' age and the number of sounds in the inventory. Despite this variation, a number of constraints emerged from an analysis of distinctions (statable as features) rather than sounds per se. All 34 inventories could be assigned to one of five typological and implicationally related levels of complexity as shown in (4).

(4) Typology of Pretreatment Phonetic Inventories for Thirty-Four Misarticulating Children

Level A: [syllabic], [consonantal], [sonorant], [coronal]

Subject 4:	b	d		
	m	n	ŋ	
	w		j	ʔh

Level B: [voice]

Subject 26:	pb	td	kg	
	m	n	ŋ	
	w		j	ʔh

Level C: [continuant], [delayed release]

Subject 13:	pb	td	kg	Subject 8:	pb	td	kg
	fv				fv	sz	ʃ
	m	n	ŋ			ts dz	čǰ
	w	j	ʔh		m	n	ŋ
					w	j	h

Level D: [nasal]

Subject 15:	pb	td	kg	Subject 36:	pb	td	kg
	fv	θð	ʃ			sz ʃ	
		čǰ					
	m	n	ŋ		m	n	
		l				r	
	w	j	ʔ		w	j	ʔh

Level E: [strident], [lateral]

Subject 39:	pb	td	kg	Subject 17:	pb	td	kg
	fv θð	sz	ʃ		fv	sz	ʃ
		čǰ				ts	čǰ
	m	n	ŋ		m	n	ŋ
		l				l	r
	w	j	ʔh		w	j	ʔ

Each inventory could be described as a set of sounds specified by a limited set of distinctive features (Chomsky and Halle 1968). The simplest type of inventory, Level A, was limited to nasals, glides, and obstruent stops, with no voice contrast among the obstruents. The major class features and a place of articulation feature were sufficient to describe Level A inventories. Level B inventories only added a voice distinction among the stops. Level C inventories added a manner distinction such that fricatives and/or affricates occurred. Thus, some inventories included stops and fricatives but no affricates. Other inventories included stops and affricates but no fricatives. Still others included stops, fricatives, and affricates. Level D inventories were characterized by the inclusion of one liquid consonant (either [l] or [r]) along with all distinctions associated with simpler inventories. Finally, Level E inventories were characterized by a stridency distinction (i.e., [s] vs. [θ]) and/or a laterality distinction (i.e., [r] vs. [l]), along with all distinctions associated with simpler levels.

This characterization specifies a series of implicational relationships among classes of sounds constituting phonetic inventories. Specifically, a stridency or laterality distinction in an inventory implies a nasal/nonnasal distinction (among sonorant consonants), which in turn implies a manner distinction (either [continuant] or [delayed release]), which implies a voice distinction, which implies a place of articulation distinction ([coronal]) and the major class distinctions ([consonantal], [sonorant] and [syllabic]).

These cross sectional characteristics of disordered phonetic inventories were found to correspond with cross sectional and longitudinal characteristics of normal first acquired phonetic inventories. A review of the research literature reveals that stops, nasals, and glides (Level A) are among the first acquired sounds and that the stridency and laterality distinctions (Level E) are acquired late (see Stoel-Gammon and Dunn 1985 for a review). For example, Leopold's (1947) diary study of Hildegard revealed that she exhibited a Level A inventory around the age of 1 year. Also, Vihman, Ferguson, and Elbert (1986) provided a detailed cross sectional investigation of individual differences in the phonetic inventories of seven young children at the 15-word stage. All of their subjects exhibited inventories that could be assigned to one of the levels of complexity presented in (4). Specifically, levels B, C, and D were evidenced.

From these results, it appears that the phonetic inventories of speech disordered systems are governed by severe constraints and that these constraints appear to be the same constraints that govern normal first acquired inventories. As a further test of this claim, Dinnsen, Chin, and Elbert (1992), in a follow-up study, examined the post-treatment phonetic inventories of the subjects from the original study (Dinnsen et al. 1990). Three sounds had been targeted for treatment in a conventional minimal pair contrast treatment program. The results of the follow-up study are summarized in (5).

(5) Typology of Posttreatment Phonetic Inventories for Thirty-Four Misarticulating Children

Level A: [syllabic], [consonantal], [sonorant], [coronal]

Subject 4:	b	d	g
	m	n	ŋ
	w	j	ʔh

Level B: [voice]

(No examples)

Level C: [continuant], [delayed release]

Subject 26:	pb	td	kg	Subject 27:	pb	td	
	fv	θð			f	sz	ʃ
	m	n	ŋ				čǰ
	w	j	ʔh		m	n	
					w	j	ʔh

Level D: [nasal]

Subject 16:			
	pb	td	k
	fv		
	m	n	ŋ
		l	
	w	j	h

Level E: [strident], [lateral]

Subject 15:				Subject 11:			
	pb	td	kg		pb	td	kg
	fv	θð sz	ʃ		fv	sz	ʃ
		čǰ				čǰ	
	m	n	ŋ		m	n	ŋ
		l				l r	
	w	j	ʔh		w	j	ʔh

All inventories changed following treatment. Some sounds were lost from inventories, and others were added. The sounds added were not always those treated, and the sounds treated were not always added. Despite this variation, one striking principle emerged. All changes in the phonetic inventories conformed with the constraints governing cross-sectional variation. This means that all post-treatment inventories could be assigned uniquely to one of the established levels of complexity. The power of this principle is especially evident in those relatively simple inventories that changed to a more complex inventory and acquired the implicationally related distinctions without direct treatment on those sounds.

The discovery of these laws derived from the conventional application of linguistic theory. The characterization of disordered systems embodied in these laws is important to both linguistic theory and speech pathology. The variation evident in the phonetic inventories of this population is highly principled and perfectly consistent with variation in normally developing systems. Given that there is nothing deviant about disordered systems, then, the variation evident in these systems is relevant to theories of language variation and change. The clinical significance of these implicational laws is that they predetermine the course of change that can occur with or without treatment. They also have implications in intervention for the selection of treatment targets, because treatment directed at the most marked (or complex) distinction (e.g., stridency) should entail or enhance the acquisition of less marked distinctions without direct treatment on those properties of inventories.

The results of our research program reveal disordered systems to be highly varied. The variation, however, is not unlimited. In fact, it appears to be quite principled. Moreover, the principles governing disordered systems do not appear to differ from those governing developing or established systems. The disordered systems we investigated represent a principled variety of natural language and of English in particular. While these disordered systems differ from one another and from English in certain respects, they all do resemble English in various ways. The resemblances are attributable to the constraints that govern all language systems and the selective attention of the acquirer on a prominent but independent property of the phonology. All linguistic constraints allow for variation within the limits of that constraint. The variation associated with the disordered systems was within the allowable limits of those constraints. The relative independence of the various properties of phonology contribute to even greater variation. For example, the lexicon may increase in size (number of words), but the number of phonological distinctions may remain relatively few. The acquisition process appears to be a matter of attention or focus on a particular property of the phonology. One child may focus his attention on achieving correct phonetic representations and formulate hypotheses that are wrong but still derive some correct productions. Another child may focus his attention on correctly internalizing underlying representations even if some errors occur at the phonetic level. Phonological rules of various types may be constructed to mediate between levels of representation that may or may not be correct. These rules must, however, comply both functionally and substantively with the constraints governing phonological rules in primary languages.

What is called a disorder may be nothing more than the 'small shoe' phenomenon. A child's foot has outgrown a now tight shoe. This may result in some discomfort for the child, and it may even cause the child to walk funny. But the shoe is still wearable, and the shoe is still one of the possible shoes that are available to children. The child's funny walking is still recognized as walking. The child's foot is still a foot that conforms to all the laws governing feet. Buying a bigger shoe might eliminate the distinguishing symptoms, but the shoe must still conform to the constraints governing shoes. Buying a shoe that is too big will not cause the foot to grow bigger, but it may cause other symptoms of another sort to arise. It is quite likely that at one time or another, we have all worn shoes that did not fit. Shoes and feet define us all. The fit is more or less good. Likewise, the grammar (phonology) of any language is a shoe that fits one person better than another. A language is thus a distribution of systems around the mean. The fit of any one system with the mean is more or less good. The so-called disordered systems fit less well with the mean. The extent to which they depart from the mean, however, provides some clues about the nature and independence of the various components or properties of grammar. This conception of the nature of language demands that linguists consider descriptions of disordered systems in the construction and testing of linguistic theory. Even greater insights about the nature of human language may derive from the investigation of disorders because of the possibilities of experimental manipulation that naturally present themselves through experimental treatment studies in the clinic.

Notes

*We would like to thank Phil Connell, Fred Eckman, Mary Elbert, and Judith Gierut for their comments and suggestions on this paper and throughout the course of the research summarized here.

This work was supported in part by grants to Indiana University from the National Institutes of Health (NS20976 and DC00260).

1. Such a possibility was first noted by Fred Eckman (personal communication) in his description of the interlanguage of a native Spanish speaker. This speaker produced the word 'smoother' correctly with the target appropriate voiced interdental fricative in word-medial position. While this word was produced correctly, the morphophonemically related form 'smooth' was pronounced incorrrectly as [smut]. The alternation was accounted for by a word final devoicing rule and an intervocalic spirantization rule. These rules operated on the incorrect underlying representation /smud/ to yield both correct and incorrect phonetic representations.

References

Adjemian, C. 1976. "On the Nature of Interlanguage Systems". *Language Learning* 26.297-320.

Camarata, S. and J. Gandour. 1984. "On Describing Idiosyncratic Phonologic Systems". *Journal of Speech and Hearing Disorders* 49.262-266.

Chomsky, N., and M. Halle. 1968. *The Sound Pattern of English*. New York: Harper & Row.

Crystal, D. 1980. *An Introduction to Language Pathology*. London: Edward Arnold.

Dinnsen, D.A. and S.B. Chin. 1988. "Linguistic and Clinical Aspects of Functional Speech Disorders". Paper presented at the Annual Meeting of the Linguistic Society of America, New Orleans.

Dinnsen, D.A., S.B. Chin, and M. Elbert. 1992. "On the Lawfulness of Change in Phonetic Inventories". *Lingua* 86. 207-222.

Dinnsen, D.A., S.B. Chin, M. Elbert, and T.W. Powell. 1990. "Some Constraints on Functionally Disordered Phonologies: Phonetic Inventories and Phonotactics. *Journal of Speech and Hearing Research* 33.28-37.

Dinnsen, D.A. and M. Elbert. 1984. "On the Relationship between Phonology and Learning". *Phonological Theory and the Misarticulating Child (ASHA Monographs Number 22)* ed. by M. Elbert, D.A. Dinnsen, and G. Weismer, 59-68. Rockville, MD: American Speech-Language-Hearing Association.

Dinnsen, D.A. and E.M. Maxwell. 1981. "Some Phonology Problems from Functional Misarticulators". *Innovations in Linguistics Education* 2:1.79-98.

Eckman, F.R. 1987. "On the Naturalness of Interlanguage Phonological Rules". *Interlanguage Phonology: The Acquisition of a Second Language Sound System* ed. by G. Ioup and S.H. Weinberger, 125-144. Cambridge, MA: Newbury House.

Gierut, J.A. 1986. "Sound Change: A Phonemic Split in a Misarticulating Child". *Applied Psycholinguistics* 7.57-68.

Gierut, J.A., M. Elbert, and D.A. Dinnsen. 1987. "A Functional Analysis of Phonological Knowledge and Generalization Learning in Misarticulating Children". *Journal of Speech and Hearing Research* 30.462-479.

Houlihan, K. and G.K. Iverson. 1979. "Functionally-Constrained Phonology. *Current Approaches to Phonological Theory* ed. by D.A. Dinnsen, 50-73. Bloomington, IN: Indiana University Press.

Ingram, D. 1976. *Phonological Disability in Children*. New York: American Elsevier Publishing Company.

Ingram, D. 1981. *Procedures for the Phonological Analysis of Children's Language*. Baltimore: University Park Press.

Leopold, W.F. 1947. *Speech Development of a Bilingual Child: A Linguist's Record. Volume II: Sound-learning in the First Two Years*. Evanston, IL: Northwestern University.

Selinker, L. 1972. "Interlanguage". *International Review of Applied Linguistics* 10.209-231.

Shibatani, M. 1972. "The Phonological Representations of English Inflectional Endings". *Glossa* 6.117-127.

Stoel-Gammon, C. and C. Dunn. 1985. *Normal and Disordered Phonology in Children*. Baltimore, MD: University Park Press.

Vihman, M.M., C.A. Ferguson, and M. Elbert. 1986. "Phonological Development from Babbling to Speech: Common Tendencies and Individual Differences". *Applied Psycholinguistics* 7.3-40.

Weismer, G., D.A. Dinnsen, and M. Elbert. 1981. "A Study of the Voicing Distinction Associated with Omitted, Word-final Stops. *Journal of Speech and Hearing Disorders* 40.320-328.

Williams, A.L. and D.A. Dinnsen. 1987. "A Problem of Allophonic Variation in a Speech Disordered Child". *Innovations in Linguistics Education* 5:1.85-90.

Applying Linguistic Theory to Clinical Language Teaching

Phil J. Connell
Indiana University

The past several years have seen a renewal in interest in developing and testing theories of language acquisition spurred mostly by Chomsky's (1981, 1986a, 1986b) remarkable theory of Universal Grammar (UG). Researchers in child language acquisition have become actively engaged in projects to describe and explain the process by which children acquire language (Hyams 1987; Guilfoyle and Noonan 1988; Kazman 1988; Lebeaux 1987). This represents a radical change from the activities of child language researchers from as little as five years ago when the emphasis was on finding better ways to describe but not explain stages of development (e.g. Brown 1973) or on searching for the cues in motherese that might correspond to these descriptive stages (Snow 1978). The explanations for language acquisition were being sought outside of the language faculty, either in general cognitive development of the child or in the structured input of the caregiver. No concerted effort was being made to explain the process from within the context of the language faculty itself (Atkinson 1987; Pinker 1984). One of the reasons for this is that the most influential theory of the language faculty, Generative Theory, paid so little attention to the process of language acquisition. Chomsky (1965) claimed that acquisition was essentially an instantaneous process once the learner performed some rather cursory analysis of the input language. The recent change in Generative Theory has made it more accessible to researchers because it offers testable claims about the details of the acquisition process. Testing these claims has led to some important new insights in the process of language acquisition and the nature of human language.

In contrast, the theory shift has had little or no impact on the day-to-day clinical language teaching that is performed in our public schools and in private and public clinics by Speech-Language Pathologists. Clinical teaching methods have traditionally been organized around descriptions of normal acquisition to convey the content of teaching lessons, that is, the goals of a lesson and the sequence by which the goals are addressed. In essence, Speech-Language Pathologists have displayed the same reluctance to refer to a linguistic theory to conceptualize teaching methods as have acquisition researchers and apparently for the same reasons -- a lack of clearly articulated explanation of how language is acquired. Unlike acquisition theorists, though, Speech-Language Pathologists cannot afford to ignore the issue of explanation and focus exclusively on description. The needs of their clients force them to construct a methodology of teaching, and as consequence, to appeal to some theoretical framework as a base for teaching practice. The resulting teaching approaches have been a hybrid of procedures more-or-less based on behaviorist theories of learning (e.g. Skinner 1957) and empiricists' descriptions of acquisition (Bloomfield 1933; Brown 1973; Maratsos 1982). The tradition of language teaching in SLP can be characterized as a set of common-sense procedures that were constructed in response to a practical need to help children but having no coherent connection to a logical explanation of how languages are acquired naturally.

Given the inadequacies of the traditional approaches to teaching and the recent change in the direction of acquisition research, it should not be long before generative theory has a substantial impact on clinical language teaching. The theory has potentially much to offer a SLP because it gives a clinician the capacity to make specific claims about how a learner initially acquires a grammar and how the grammar changes into an adult grammar. Thus, a teacher who applies the theory has a principled method for determining what to teach, how to teach and what to expect as an outcome.

This chapter will describe some preliminary attempts along the lines of constructing teaching methodologies that model these new explanations of language acquisition. The students who are the recipients of the teaching that will be described are an identifiable group of children who have had great difficulty acquiring language even though they have none of the cognitive or perceptual impairments that are known to hinder language learning. They are called Specific Language Impaired (SLI) to signify the fact that their developmental problem appears to be specific to language learning (Rosenberg 1984). In experiments that will be described, groups of these children have been taught aspects of language using experimentally controlled teaching approaches that implement certain claims about theories of language acquisition. These teaching experiments have provided information that may lead to an understanding of the conditions that underlie the language learning disorder, the similarity between language-impaired and normal children, and the nature of the early languages of abnormal and normal children.

The preponderance of evidence that has been gathered to date on SLI children indicates that they have difficulty acquiring language with the ease of normal children but that the initial and intermediate languages that they acquire on the way to acquiring the adult language are the same as those of normal children (see Leonard 1987, for a thorough review of the evidence). Thus, SLI children appear to learn the same language in the same way as normal children except that the onset of acquisition is later, the rate of acquisition is slower, and the final level of achievement is lower. Their problem is apparently one of speed of movement through the same intermediate languages that normal children pass through on their way to acquiring the adult language. The alternative but unattested model is one in which the grammars of SLI children are unusual in some crucial aspect, for example, they could contain computational rules that are not found or in the grammars of unafflicted children. There is no evidence that this is the case. Thus, from the data that is presently available, the more likely scenario is that SLI children take an overly protracted time to acquire a language.

The research that will be described focuses on learning grammars that generate simple sentences. Some of the work has concerned learning meanings that are encoded by means of the syntax of simple sentences and other part concerns the acquisition of derivational morphology. The overall purpose of this work has been to examine the question of whether SLI children learn language differently from normal children.

Some sentences that are typical of SLI children are depicted in Table 1. As a general description of the abridged sample of the three children present, it can be said that these sentences could have been spoken by children who are as much as two years younger. The sample of the first child contains no utterances of longer than one word. There is no evidence in this or the longer sample from which these utterances are taken that indicates that the child knows the syntactic functions of sentences. The utterances of the second child generally contain no NP in the subject position. It might be hypothesized that the grammar that generates these sentences contain no specification for the subject position if it were not for sentences such as the

Table 1. Representative samples of SLI children's utterances

Child 1 Age: 3:9	Child 2 Age: 4:2	Child 2 Age: 4:2
This.	Eat this.	Me holding.
Mine.	Boy.	This Tracy.
Doggy.	Go home?	This say Tracy.
This?	Reading people.	It mine.
Big.	Me hanging on shirt.	I going somewhere after this.

last in which an accusative case pronoun appears in what appears to be the subject position.

The sentences of the third child indicate a grammar that is more advanced but still is quite different from an adult grammar. The utterances all contain material in the subject position but the morphemes associated with the subject of sentences, that is, agreement morphology for person and number, are missing or are improperly used.

The teaching research that has been performed on this type of child has generally concerned testing hypotheses that emanate from two models of language teaching that correspond to two models of language acquisition. The first is an induction model. It contains a learning component that recognizes patterns in the input data and a hypothesis-making component that proposes a rule that captures the pattern . There is some disagreement about whether this kind of learning can be logically free of innate language knowledge (e.g. Atkinson 1987). Some hold that the learner has constraints on the patterns that are pursued in the input and the kinds of hypotheses that can be generated and others would disagree with this characterization. Following the lead of Bloomfield, some hold that the process is completely unguided and follows learning principles that are part of a general cognitive faculty (e.g. Maratsos 1982). Following the lead of Chomsky, others hold that only those patterns that are found in natural languages can be explored and only those rules that are found can be hypothesized (e.g. Hyams 1987).

The second model is a deduction model. In this model, the learner is guided by a set of principles of language that constrain the kinds of grammars that can be learned and by a set of parameters that allow for the kinds of variation that may occur among languages. Following the thinking of Chomsky, acquisition is conceptualized as a series of grammars that are consecutively reorganized until a steady state grammar is attained. Each of the grammars in the sequence conforms to the principles of UG and each of the reorganizations is either a product of a trigger that resets a parameter or of the maturation of a principle that was not available at an earlier biological stage.

An induction methodology has been used to teach certain aspects of language to SLI children (Connell 1986a). The methodology is essentially one of structuring the input sentences in such a way as to clearly depict the the relation between form and meaning. In one study, the rule taught was one of structuring the input sentences in such a way as to clearly depict the relation between form and meaning. In one study, the rule taught was stage of development. They were taught in a single-subject experimental design to ensure that the effects of learning were the product of the teaching program and not from an external source. The children were taught using pairs of pictures depicting cartoon characters who were engaged in an activity such as pushing each other across the floor on a wagon. The pusher (agent) and pushee (patient) roles are reversed in the two pictures. By providing the children with simple sentences describing the actions depicted in the pictures, the learner is led to interpret the relation between word order and thematic roles. After being presented with such data in a structured teaching format, the children were able to correctly select from different pairs of pictures based on the thematic roles of sentences describing them and were able to say sentences in which NPs representing the referents portraying the thematic roles were appropriately ordered. It is not clear what the children actually learned from the contrast but it is clear that they were not using such sequences of words prior to the teaching program and that they were unable to interpret the meaning of such sentences. The question of what was learned is the same as the question of what they knew about language before the teaching began. Neither of these questions can be satisfactorily answered as of yet but the methodology of teaching and testing offers an avenue for addressing them.

Besides indicating that the teaching methodology modeled after theoretical accounts of acquisition can be successful in teaching at least some aspect of language to these children, it also provides a clue to the etiology of the language learning disorder. The SLI children needed to imitate the reversible sentences in order to learn. When the teaching strategy consisted of merely asking them to point to the correct picture to interpret a given sentence, the subjects did not learn to identify the correct picture nor to say sentences. When, on the other hand, they were asked to imitate a sentence describing a picture and then say the sentence on their own, they were successful at learning. Whatever they may have learned from the process, learning only occurred from imitating sentence pairs corresponding to reversible pictures.

This finding has generated a series of subsequent studies concerned with determining whether the facilitating effects of imitation are unique to SLI children (Connell 1987, Roseberry and Connell, 1991). In a later study (Connell 1987) an invented suffixal morpheme was taught to both SLI and normal children to determine if they differed in terms of their reaction to imitation teaching. Forty SLI and age-matched normals were taught that the suffix /a/ meant "part of" such that car-a meant part of a car. This derivational morpheme is not part of English but there is a similar morpheme in German, for example, autoteil means part of a car. Half of the children in each group were taught the morpheme by merely listening to an adult recite the name of a whole object (e.g., bell) and a part of an object (e.g. bella) while pointing to pictures whole and then part-objects. The other half had the added requirement of repeating the adults' naming of both kinds of pictures. The children in both conditions were presented with 20 words to which the morpheme was appended.

What emerged from the study was a pattern of learning that clearly differentiates SLI children. The SLI children learned much faster if they said (repeated) the noun + suffix while the normal children learned faster when hearing the adult say the names and learned slower when they had to repeat the adult's words. This pattern of learning has been confirmed in a recent experiment in which Spanish-speaking children who were learning English as a second language were identified as SLI by their unusual inability to learn the invented morpheme through observation (Roseberry and Connell forthcoming). This line of research is being pursued in a series of studies. The question that is being pursued is whether the superiority of imitation learning is a reflection of their general cognitive faculties or is isolated to language learning.

In summary, it appears that SLI children have difficulty making generalizations about input data unless they are forced to imitate it. Imitation is an unusual and unnatural teaching procedure that seems to facilitate the induction process of SLI children. It is unusual because it does not facilitate the process for normal children placed in the same learning circumstances and it is unnatural in that it does not appear to play much of a role in the normal language acquisition process (Berko Gleason 1988).

Any reasoned analysis of the process of induction teaching will come to the conclusion that there is a serious limitation to what can be taught by the approach. The limitation is that rules that express a rather direct relation between meaning and utterance, such as theta role and lexical teaching and in teaching certain morphemes, especially the derivational ones like the invented one from above, can be taught. Morphemes need not be derivational as long as their function correlates with a semantic distinction. The plural morpheme is a good example of an inflectional morpheme that fits this mold. Its meaning — more than one — and its form — a suffix — can be taught through physical demonstration because there is a strong correlation between meaning and form. Pictures of a group of objects can be contrasted with pictures of single objects to demonstrate that the suffix corresponds to a distinct meaning.

The distinctions within the pronoun case system in English is an example of a part of language that can not fit into the induction teaching scheme. The contrast between the nominative and accusative cases, as exemplified in the following sequence, *This is Gloria. Here, she is kissing a man. Now, the man is kissing her* illustrate the abstract nature of pronoun case. If a child were taught that the change in reference to Gloria from she to her was related to the thematic role the NPs played in the respective sentences, the child would have been given erroneous information about case in English. Using the terminology of the theory of UG, nominative case is said to be assigned by abstract tense part of INFL, a point that will be clarified later, which is quite independent of the thematic role played by the NP. Such an abstraction appears to be well beyond the capacity of induction teaching because the rules in question have no possibility of physical demonstration. That is, no picture or other type of demonstration could facilitate the teaching of the she-her contrast.

The limitation that plagues the induction teaching is the same that plagues any theory of language that does not allow for innate language knowledge to direct the kinds of inductions that a learner makes. The problem is explaining how children make just the right inductions given that the right ones (such as pronoun case) are abstract and not obvious if such innate information is not operating. A teaching procedure that is constructed on the assumption that such innate information is available has been implemented in an experimental teaching study (Connell 1986b). One drawback to performing such research is that theoretical accounts of language acquisition are rapidly evolving even within the UG framework.

Applying any aspect of them to teaching is undoubtedly a bit premature. This position, though, seems to be a bit too conservative for two reasons. First, the approaches presently taken to teaching abstract syntax have not been shown to be effective. There is no rich tradition of successful teaching that would argue against using experimental and tenuous methods. Secondly, the outcome of such teaching methods with SLI children, children who appear to learn language in the same manner as normal children only more slowly, may provide important data for developing theories of acquisition in general. That is, hypotheses generated from theoretical accounts can be tested with teaching data and the theories can be modified accordingly.

The study in question concerned a pattern of language errors that most SLI children display once their language learning progresses into sentences. This pattern is reflected in the third child's data in Table 1. Table 2 contains a longer sample of the same subject. Table 3 contains a list of the properties that characterize the samples of such children.

The characteristics listed in Table 3 have been the concern of a group of people who are attempting to characterize the Null Subject parameter in

Table 2. A sample of sentences spoken by a SLI child

Utterance	Guide to Interpretation
What is this?	Topic: toy car
All done?	Topic: teaching session
In there?	Topic: Toy car
See Mommy.	(I want to see Mommy)
Put it on him.	Topic: self
Ben need this car.	
Right to Ben.	Topic: my car
Pick up the dirt.	Topic: toy truck

Table 3. Lists of properties commonly found in language samples of SLI children

Missing Subject NP
Missing auxiliary BE
Missing copula
Missing third-person, singular, indicative
Missing infinitive TO
Substitution of accusative for nominative case pronouns
No question inversion

theoretical work on normal children's language. A parameter within the GB framework is analogous to a switch that the language learner sets in response to certain input data called triggers. The process of language acquisition has been characterized as a process of setting a series of parameters creating a series of grammars that eventually lead to a steady state adult grammar (Hyams 1987). In the case of the Null Subject parameter, there are several proposed triggers and several proposals about the nature of the parameter itself (Hyams 1987; Guilfoyle and Noonan 1988; Kazman 1988, Lebeaux 1987). The parameter was originally proposed to characterize the regular difference between languages concerning whether they allow a sentence without overt subjects. For example in English, the sentence **Am a walrus* is agrammatical but the equivalent sentence in Italian *Sono il tricheco* is grammatical, thus Italian allows (overtly) subjectless sentences and English does not. Child English appears to have a grammar that allows null subjects in a manner that is similar in some ways to Chinese rather than Italian in that the Chinese does not have the elaborate agreement morphology of Italian. The language characteristics listed in Table 3 appear to be in the domain of this parameter because certain natural languages that allow subjectless sentences also have these characteristics. Interestingly, it appears that normal English-speaking children begin to use overt subjects at the same time that they acquire these other elements (Hyams 1987). Thus, it appears possible to characterize the grammar of SLI children at this stage as one that differs from the adult grammar in terms of the Null Subject parameter as well as other aspects of grammar. This characterization leads to a teaching approach that will be described shortly.

Before discussing how the setting the parameter might be addressed in a teaching program, some ground has to be covered concerning the structure of sentences containing different kinds of NPs serving as the subject of adult English sentences and of other languages. The sentence in Figure 1 is an example. In *John is walking the dog*, the subject *John* is a type of NP called an r-expression in GB. Among other possible reasons, one might use the proper noun *John* to refer to John, as opposed to a pronoun such as he, in order to introduce John as the topic of the ensuing discourse. One of the functions of r-expressions is to create a new discourse topic. If John were already the discourse topic, reference to him would best be accomplished by the pronominal he, a second type of NP. The fact that the discourse topic is other than John (thus making John allowable as the referring expression) is specified by the term "unspecified" in the discourse topic slot

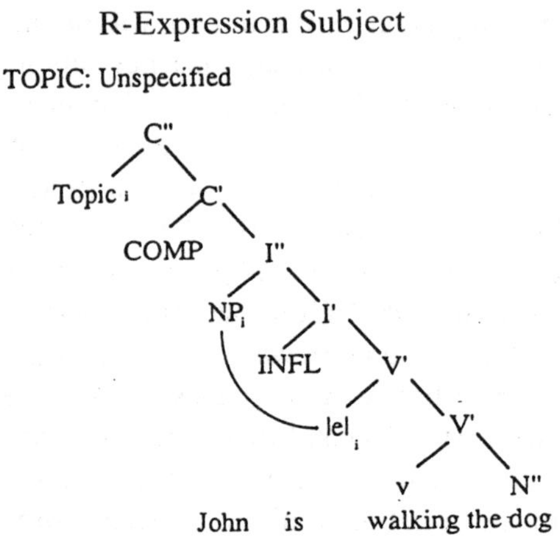

Figure 1. Tree representation of an r-expression subject

(indicated as TOPIC above the tree) in Figure 1. The tree used to describe the structure of this sentence uses the notation of extended X-bar theory with the addition of the Koopman and Sportiche (1987) stipulation that subject NPs are raised from the specifier of the VP to the specifier of the IP for case assignment and other things. The CP contains an NP position that will be called the sentence topic (the specifier position and indicated as Topic) after Huang (1984). The sentence topic is what the sentence is about while the discourse topic is what the conversation is about at any one point. What is important to note about this tree description is the NP that is the subject of the sentence is not referring to nor is it coindexed with the discourse topic. The sentence topic is coindexed with the subject as indicated by the subscripted i. That is, the sentence can be said to be about the person whose name (proper noun) is the subject of the sentence but whose identity is not what the discourse is about. These conditions set the stage for an noun like John to be the subject of the sentence.

The relation between the subject, the sentence Topic and the discourse TOPIC is different when a pronoun is allowed to serve as the subject of a sentence as illustrated in Figure 2. What is different in this case is that they are all coindexed, that is, they all refer to the person John. The conversation at this point is about John, this sentence is a comment about John that fits into the ongoing discourse and the subject of the sentence is an NP that

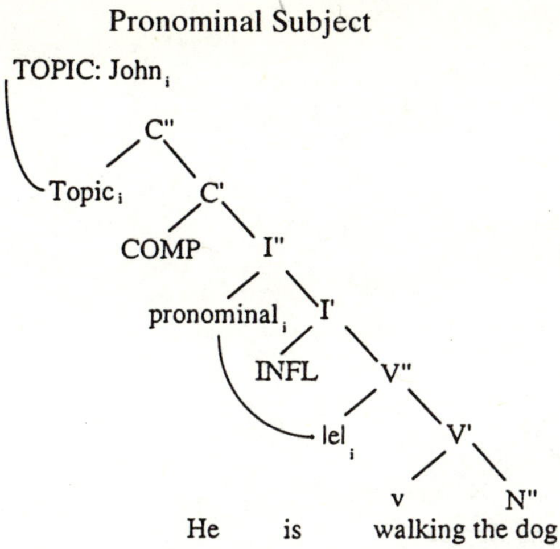

Figure 2. Tree representation of a pronominal subject

refers to John. These conditions dictate that the subject NP to be realized as a pronominal. Thus, one of the conditions that allow subject pronominal reference in English is a three-way coindexing of the two topics and the subject.

Some languages like Italian allow for the generation of an NP type called pro rather than a pronominal in situations where three-way coindexing occurs. Such languages have been called Pro-Drop Languages to indicate that the subject pronoun may be dropped from the surface sentence. This situation is illustrated in Figure 3. A pro is projected from the IP node. The pro has all the characteristics of an overt NP except that it has no phonetic realization, that is, it is silent. Even though the subject is unsaid, understanding the reference of the pro is as unambiguous for an Italian listener as is understanding the reference of a pronominal for an English speaker listening to the sentence described in Figure 2. Reference is said to be chained to the discourse topic. In the Italian case, there is agreement morphology attached to the verb that can help identify the person and number of the person referred to by pro, in this case as a third person singular suffix. This morphological information appears to be redundant because in some languages, such as Chinese, such morphological information is not available and the identification of the referent of pro is not a problem. The discourse topic is identified as the referent.

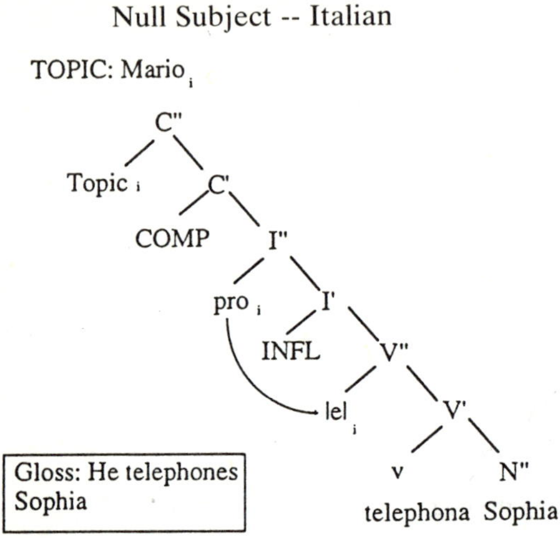

Figure 3. Tree representation of an Italian pro subject

Thus, English and Italian are said to differ parametrically in their use of subject pronominals or pro in situations where there is three-way coindexing. The parameter that differentiates them is called the Null Subject parameter. The purpose of the parameter from a learner's perspective is to specify whether the grammar that is being constructed will allow pro in the subject position. There is some dispute over whether all instances of null subjects in early child language are actually the result of missetting this parameter for English or of a lack of maturation of other aspects of grammar. Hyams (1987) proposes that it is a function of a missetting. She claims that the default setting of the parameter allows pro in subject position of all child languages. Kazman (1988), Lebeaux (1987) and Guilfoyle and Noonan (1988), on the other hand, propose that the missing subjects are a product of early grammars that do not have a subject NP node specified. Without such a node, the subject NP would not be generated which would explain the missing subjects without appealing to the machinery of parameters. Kazman argues that the Null Subject parameter becomes involved later in acquisition after the grammar obtains more of the characteristics of the adult grammar. That is, the grammar has to first project a subject NP node before a parameter that involves it can be addressed.

The distinction between the two hypotheses is basically a difference in theories about the nature of the force that drives children to abandon grammars and adopt new ones on their way toward the steady state grammar. Hyams claims that the force for change lies in the triggering of parameters. When a child attends to the data that is critical to triggering a parameter, the parameter will be set and the grammar will change. The others mentioned are skeptical that the force for change is solely data-driven and follow Borer and Wexler's (1987) logic that certain UG principles become available only as the learner matures. Thus, they claim that a potent force for change is the gradual attainment of deeper understandings of the nature of language that comes with biological maturity.

The distinction between the early grammars that are proposed from these two hypotheses is presented in Figures 4 and 5. As depicted in left and right side of Figure 4, the grammar proposed by Hyams has much of the complexity as an adult grammar[1] although some of the detail of the INFL node is missing. There is no tense, agreement or auxiliary projections in the head of INFL. As indicated, Subject NPs may or may not be null. They are not null when they are not coindexed with the discourse topic, as in the adult grammar of English and Italian, as depicted in the left side of Figure 4. They are null when they are coindexed as in the grammar of Italian, as depicted in the right side of Figure 5. The subject NP of this latter sentence is a pro that is coindexed with the sentence and discourse topic. In actuality, she claims the process of identifying the referent for pro in this grammar is more like Chinese because it, like early child English, lacks the rich agreement morphology of languages like Italian. The occasional emergence of pronominals in what appears to be subject position is claimed to be, in actuality, a topic pronoun projected from the sentence topic node, not the subject NP node. Thus, it does not receive nominative (subject) case. By changing the default setting of the Null Subject parameter to the setting that is appropriate for English, a child disallows pro as a possible projection of the subject NP. The proposed process that leads to this change in setting will be discussed below.

As depicted in Figure 6, the Kazman (1988) model, the grammar is severely underspecified compared to the grammar that will emerge once the child matures. What is most noticeably missing is the INFL node (IP). Kazman claims that what others have taken as evidence for an INFL node, namely, the use of suffixes such as the progressive *ing*, are actually base generated as morphological units affixed to the verb. The alternation

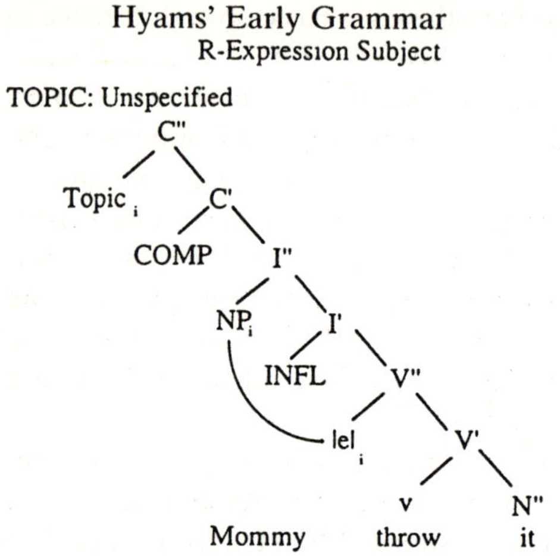

Figure 4. Tree representation of an child sentence containing an r-expression subject

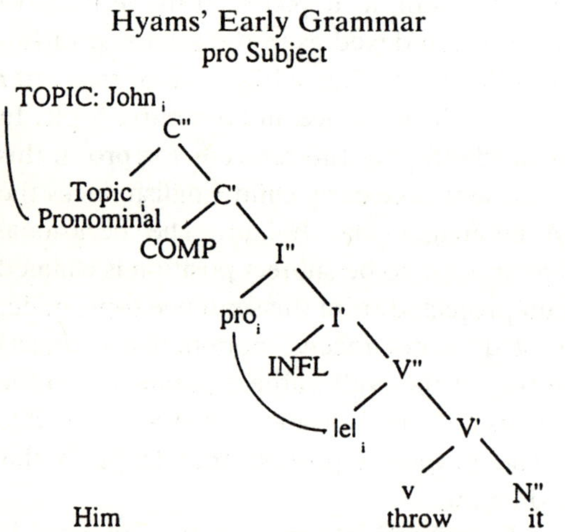

Figure 5. Tree representation of an child sentence with a pro subject

Kazman's Early Grammar

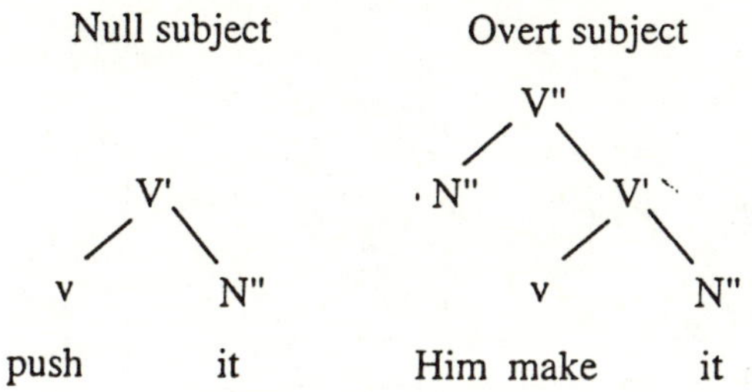

Figure 6. Tree representations of child sentences containing a null and an overt subject

between sentences containing null subjects and those that contain overt subjects is a product of a VP that projects an NP node optionally. Thus, overt and null subject sentences are base generated as such. According to Kazman's scenario, once the INFL node can be adduced, the child creates a grammar containing an obligatory NP in VP which is raised to the specifier of IP to receive case assignment. It is only after this grammar is attained can the child set the Null Subject parameter concerning the use of pro as a subject NP option.

Thus, null subjects arise from these two characterizations of early grammars from different sources. In the Hyams position, null subjects are a product of the subject NP node projecting as pro, and in the Kazman analysis, the null subjects are a consequence of the D-structure not containing a subject NP node. The two approaches are in agreement, though, on how the child eventually sets the Null Subject parameter appropriately for a given language. Kazman accepts Hyam's proposal that the parameter is set by triggers that license the use of pro in the subject NP node on the one hand and then allow the pro to be used in languages that identify null subjects properly. The conditions that relate to licensing and identifying subject pro are illustrated in the diagram in Figure 7. Licensing is a product of what Jaeggli and Safir (1989) call morphological uniformity. Languages that have uniform treatment of verbs in terms of suffixes license subject pro. That is, languages that have a rich verbal morphology such that a bare verb is not a well-formed word license subject pro as well as languages that have no verbal morphology at all. Licensing by itself, though, only allows for the

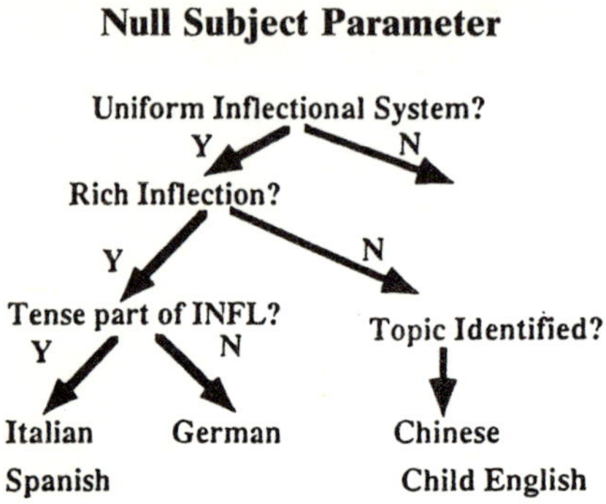

Figure 7. Licensing and identification of pro

next level of decision to be considered — whether a null subject can be properly identified. For a morphologically rich language, proper identification means that the AGR part of INFL contains TENSE, as in Italian and Spanish. Languages that have TENSE elsewhere, as in German where TENSE is claimed to be base generated in COMP, can not identify null subjects making subject pro barred. For morphologically deficient languages such as Chinese, Japanese and Korean, proper identification is based on the three-way coindexing as described previously, a chain between the subject NP node and the sentence and discourse topics.

Hyam's suggests that English speaking children's grammar licenses subject pro by having no agreement morphology (uniform) and it identifies the referent of the pro by a discourse topic chain in much the same manner as Chinese. She claims that the English learner first realizes that this grammar has to change when tense morphemes are noticed in the input data. Such data calls into question whethe subject pro can actually be licensed in the current grammar. In order the settle the issue, the learner must determine whether the verbal morphology in the input is uniform or mixed. Hyam's is not clear about how this determination is made, but perhaps the learner notices that verbs have inflections in some sentences and not in others. This leads the learner to change the grammar to one that bars subject pro. In contrast to an English learner, the Chinese learner would keep the original or default grammar because no data in the input would contradict the default setting of the parameter.

Spanish and German learners would receive contradictory data and would proceed through the same steps as the English learner until the decision concerning the uniformity of the verbal morphology is reached. Because all verbs are inflected, Spanish and German learners would make the opposite decision about uniformity, thereby retaining license for subject pro. Spanish and German learners, however, would differ in terms of the next decision to be made — whether the subject pro can be identified. The Spanish learner would decide that identification is possible because AGR and Tense are found in the INFL of the input sentences. Thus, their grammars remain the same, that is, licensing and identifying a subject pro. German learners, on the other hand, would find no Tense in the INFL of input sentences, and, as a result, change their grammar to one that bars a subject pro.

From both the maturation and the triggering perspective, English children at one point have the parameter set the wrong way. This is the constant state for the Hyams' child and a state of later development for the Kazman child. Assuming the validity of this characterization, the question of importance to teachers of SLI children is how to reset the parameter. The proposed mechanism for resetting the parameter appears to be quite complex. According to all accounts, the child who has a grammar that has the wrong setting for English also has no AGR or TENSE node. Thus, it would be difficult to teach the contrast between verbs like *plays* and *played* using an induction sort of procedure outlined previously, where concepts involving the relation between the time-of-event and the time-of-speech (e.g. *he walks* versus *he walked*) the recurrence of an event (e.g. *he is walking to work* versus *he walks to work*) is demonstrated by pictures or physical enactments. If the learner did not have a means for representing the TENSE and AGR material available in the input sentences, there is no reason to expect that an analysis of these elements could be used to reset a parameter. The learner's difficulty would be complicated by the fact that AGR and TENSE is not overtly specified in all English sentences. Thus, not only would the learner have to learn about abstract elements that are not represented in the presently held grammar but would have to learn that these elements are not uniformly realized as verbal morphemes.

On the face of it, it is difficult to conceive of a teaching method that would give an SLI child the kind of input that would be needed to influence the learner in terms of licensing a subject pro and identifying its referent. The difficulty of constructing a teaching program for resetting the Null Subject parameter is not reflected in ease by which normal children reset the parameter. They pass though a stage (more precisely, possess a grammar) that has the characteristics of a misset parameter as outlined in Table 3 during a short period of their third year of life. As indicated from the results of the experiments on the language learning capabilities of SLI children, what they need to make them learn at a more rapid pace is a teaching program that requires them to say carefully constructed sentences while observing events that represent their meanings. Given that it appears to be difficult to construct a program around those language aspects that are hypothesized to provide normal children with the data necessary to reset the parameter, a different avenue needs to be taken. The avenue that proved to be successful in a recent teaching experiment with SLI children (Connell, 1987) involved teaching children a set of sentences that led them to abandon there Null Subject grammar for a grammar that did not allow null subjects. The teaching procedure emanated from what can be called the Brute Force Hypothesis. The assumption underlying the hypothesis is that teaching that is directed towards resetting a parameter for an SLI child may need to be fundamentally different from the natural process of resetting a parameter due to the limitations imposed by the limited context of teaching and the limited capabilities of the learner. The hypothesis predicts that teaching SLI learners to say sentences that contain elements not represented in their grammar will cause them to reorganize their grammar to accommodate the elements if and only if the reorganization required is parametric. It is predicted that learners of this type will reset a parameter as a result of learning to represent sentences that could not be represented under their presently held grammar. This process of grammatical change is proposed only under conditions that are within the domain of a parameter. This, then, is a process of resetting that is the reverse of that which is typically proposed in normal acquisition.

This hypothesis was tested in a teaching study involving four SLI children (ages 3:5 to 4:2) who were using either null, an r-expression or an accusative pronominal in the subject position of their sentences as illustrated in Table 4. The samples of these children were similar to that of the child whose sample is depicted in Table 2. The teaching procedure involved the children saying sentences that contained two overt pronominals in the preverbal position such as in her, *she is petting the fawn*. The one of the two pronouns in this sentence could not be represented in a grammar that allowed null subjects as characterized by Hyams. According to Hyams (see

Table 4. Different kinds of NP in the subject position of sentences spoken by a group of SLI children

Example Sentence:	Overt NP type
(I) Put it on him.	Null (pro)
Him put it.	Accusative Pronoun (pronominal)
Ben need this car.	Own name (r-expression)
Dinosaur hiding.	Noun (r-expression)

Figure 5), one preverbal pronoun of a sentence would be interpreted as the sentence topic and the second would have obtain no interpretation because there is only one overt slot available. Thus, by teaching the children to say such sentences and to identify the referent of both pronouns, a grammar that was incompatible with that allowed by the current parameter setting was created. The intended outcome of this incompatibility is a resetting of the parameter thereby allowing such sentences to be represented.

The children were taught to represent the sentences in question by the induction approach described earlier. They were taught to say two sentence types of the form *Her, she is petting the fawn* and *She is petting the fawn* in contexts that emphasized the potential difference in their interpretation. The difference that was emphasized was the use of the accusative pronoun to unambiguously refer to a person in a crowd of people. For example, a picture depicting a crowd of people standing around a fawn and only one of them, a little girl, is petting the fawn was used to provide the children with an interpretation of the sentence with the left dislocated accusative pronoun. The teacher asked the children "Which one is petting the fawn?" and taught the children to answer "Her, she is petting the fawn" and to accompany the answer with a pointing gesture towards the girl in the picture. This situation was presented in contrast to a second picture of the same girl by herself petting the fawn. The teacher asked "What is she doing?" and taught the children to answer "She is petting the fawn". The expected effect of teaching was to make the sentence topic and subject both overt pronominals with obvious grammatical and pragmatic functions thereby teaching them to interpret a sentence that their currently held grammar could not represent. It was predicted that this would demonstrate to the children that pro need not occupy the subject position and, as a result, cause them to reset the parameter to disallow subject pro.

Table 5. Typical sentences representing the three stages of change of children taught to reset the Null Subject parameter.

Stage	*Sentence Types*
Pre-teaching	*Me going there*
	(I) Have this one
Mid-Teaching	*I going to store,*
Final Teaching	*I am going now*
	He wants one.
	Can I take it?

The results of the teaching program, which are summarized in Table 5, supported the hypothesis. The subjects began to use nominative case pronouns in the subject position of sentences spoken in conversational speech as the first indication that they were changing their grammars. According to GB, overt case marking on pronominals is assigned by the TENSE component of INFL. Thus, the use of case-marked subject pronouns is an indication that INFL specifies tense. The use of agreement morphology is an indication that the INFL also contains AGR.

There is one observation of importance about the results that calls into question whether the children underwent a complete grammatical change as a result of the teaching program. The characterization in Table 5 of the kinds of sentences children said does not include the infrequent use of sentences of the type *Him find it*. Sentences like these have been found to occur in the samples of normal children as well who appear to have acquired case and agreement previously. These two types of sentences would seem to be incompatible in that they would predict two different generating grammars. From the present perspective, a grammar that allows subject pro is different from one that does not. The two sentence types appear to represent a mixture of the new and old grammar of the children which calls into question the whole characterization of a progression of grammars. There are two possible solutions to this dilemma. The first is that children are maintaining two grammars simultaneously in much the same way that adults maintain several registers. The characterization of registers within a theory of UG has yet to be developed so the implications of this solution are entirely unknown. The second solution would allow the sentences within one grammar. The solution relates to the elision that is possible in English sentence spoken in response to questions. In response to the question "What are you doing?" might come the reply "Walking the dog". What has happened here is illustrated in Figure 9.

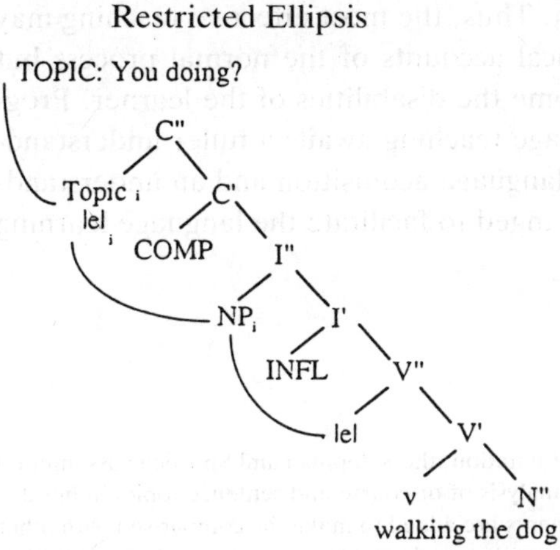

Figure 8. Tree representations of an ellipted sentence

There are other possible characterizations of this process but this seems to fit the current situation well. The missing elements are all chained to the discourse topic that is specific to the content of the question. Their elision is an indication of the redundancy of the elided material and the content of the question. What is being proposed is that these children might use this elision process but fail to honor the constraints that adults do. They may, in fact, use the process in those occasions when sentence topic is an overt pronominal. Thus, the difference between this and an adult grammar is not the use of pro vs pronominal in the subject position but on the limits placed on elision of this sort. SLI children at this stage might be said to be responding as if they were responding to unspoken questions. A fact that supports this analysis is the rare use a sentence of the form *him is running* which could be interpreted as a subject pronominal with the wrong case.

In conclusion, the studies that have been reviewed indicate that linguistic theories have much to offer researchers and clinicians who are dealing with the language learning problems of SLI children. Now that theories can be used to make specific predictions about what children learn, specific procedures can be devised to test the theory and at the same time test the effectiveness of teaching procedures. These children may not need to have the process of language acquisition revisited during teaching activities for teaching to be most effective but rather have teaching lessons that take into account their disability in learning language, that is, in making inductions about input data presented to them. Thus, the most effective teaching may be that which is based on theoretical accounts of the normal process but that modifies the process to overcome the disabilities of the learner. Progress in the clinical science of language teaching awaits a fuller understanding of the nature of the process of language acquisition and an understanding of how this process might be changed to facilitate the language learning of abnormal children.

Note

1. Hyam's did not use the extended X-bar notation, the Koopman and Sportiche assumption on subject NP raising nor the Huang analysis of discourse and sentence topics in her discussion of null subjects. These components are added to make the comparison with other characterizations clearer. These additions do not distort her proposal and are neutral to her central claims.

References

Atkinson, M. 1987. "Mechanisms for Language Acquisition: Learning, Parameter Setting and Triggering." *First Language* 7.3-30.

Bloomfield, L. 1933. *Language*. New York: Henry Holt.

Brown, R. 1973. *A First Language*. Cambridge, MA: Harvard University Press.

Berko Gleason, J. 1988. "Studying Language Development". *The Development of Language* ed. by J. Berko Gleason, 1-34. Columbus: Merrill Publishing Co.

Borer, H. and K. Wexler. 1987. "The Maturation of Syntax." Roeper and Williams 1987.123-172.

Chomsky, N. 1965. *Aspects of a Theory of Syntax*. Cambridge, MA: MIT Press.

Chomsky, N. 1981. *Lectures on Government and Binding*. Dordrecht: Foris.

Chomsky, N. 1986a. *Knowledge of Language: Its Nature, Origin and Use*. New York: Praeger.

Chomsky, N. 1986b. *Barriers*. Cambridge, MA: MIT Press.

Connell, P. 1986a. "Acquisition of Semantic Roles by Language-disordered Children: Differences between Comprehension and Production". *Journal of Speech and Hearing Research* 29.366-374.

Connell, P. 1986b. "Teaching Subjecthood to Language-disordered Children". *Journal of Speech and Hearing Research* 29.481-492.

Connell, P. 1987. "An Effect of Modeling and Imitation Teaching Procedures on Children with and without Specific Language Impairment". *Journal of Speech and Hearing Research* 30.105-113.

Huang, J. 1984. "On the Distribution and Reference of Empty Pronouns. *Linguistic Inquiry* 15. 532-573.

Hyams, N. 1987. "The Setting of the Null Subject Parameter: A Reanalysis". Paper presented and the Boston University Conference of Child Language Development, Boston, MA.

Guilfoyle, E. and M. Noonan. 1988. "Functional Categories and Language Acquisition". Paper presented and the Boston University Conference of Child Language Development, Boston, MA.

Jaeggli, O. and K. Safir. 1989. "The Null Subject Parameter and Parametric Theory". *The Null Subject Parameter* ed. by O. Jaeggli and K. Safir, 1-44. Dordrecht: Kluwer Academic Publishers.

Kazman, R. 1988. "Null Arguments and the Acquisition of Case and INFL". Paper presented and the Boston University Conference of Child Language Development, Boston, MA.

Koopman, H. and D. Sportiche. 1987. "Subjects". Unpublished manuscript, UCLA and USC.

Lebeaux, D. 1987. "Comments on Hyams". Roeper and Williams 1987.23-39.

Leonard, L. 1987. "Is Specific Language Impairment a Useful Construct?" *Advances in Applied Psycholinguistics*. Volume 1: *Disorders of First-language Development* ed. by S. Rosenberg. Cambridge: Cambridge University Press.

Maratsos, M. 1982. "The child's Construction of Grammatical Categories". *Language Acquisition: The State of the Art* ed. by E. Wanner and L. Gleitman, 240-266. Cambridge: Cambridge University Press.

Pinker, S. 1984. *Language Learnability and Language Development*. Cambridge, MA: Harvard University Press.

Roeper, T. and E. Williams, eds. 1987. *Parameter Setting*. Dordrecht: D. Reidel Publishing Co.

Rosenberg, S. 1984. "Disorders of First Language Development: Trends in Research and Theory". *Malformations in Development: Biological and Psychological Sources and Consequences* ed. by E. Gollin. New York, NY: Academic Press.

Roseberry, C. and P. Connell. 1991. "Use of an Invented Language Rule in the Differentiation of Normal and Specific-language Impaired Spanish-speaking Children". *Journal of Speech and Hearing Research* 34. 596-603.

Skinner, B. 1957. *Verbal Behavior*. Englewood Cliffs, NJ: Prentice-Hall Inc.

Snow, C. 1978. "The Conversational Context of Language Acquisition". *Recent Advances in the Psychology of Language Volume 4a*. ed. by R. Campbell and P. Smith. New York, NY: Plenum Press.

On Grammatical Deficits in Chinese Aphasia

Sylvia Chen
University of Southern California

Introduction

In studying the relationship between brain and language, two general models have been proposed for analyzing aphasic disorder: the syndrome-dominant model (Berndt and Caramazza 1980; Caramazza and Berndt 1978; Caramazza and Berndt 1985; Caramazza and Zurif 1976; Goodglass 1976; Goodglass and Menn 1985) and the language-dominant model (Bates, Friederici, and Wulfeck 1987a, 1987b; Bates, Friederici, Wulfeck, and Juarez 1988; Bates and Wulfeck 1989). The syndrome-dominant model proposes that Broca's aphasia represents a syndrome with an impairment in closed class word, by contrast, Wernicke's aphasia is a syndrome with an impairment in open class words (Berndt and Caramazza 1980; Caramazza and Berndt 1978; Caramazza and Berndt 1985; Goodglass 1976). The language-dominant model is based on the finding that the differentiation of impairments between languages is greater than the dissociation of Broca's and Wernicke's aphasia (Bates et al. 1987a, 1987b; Bates et al. 1988; MacWhinney and Osman-Sagy 1988; Smith and Bates 1987; Smith and Mimica 1984; Slobin and Talay 1988; Tzeng and Chen 1988). This model therefore predicts greater difference in aphasic syndromes across different languages than across two different syndromes.

In this paper, I am going to investigate the syndrome-dominant model and the language-dominant model through Chinese aphasics' sentence arrangement. Three typical function words and the dominant SVO word order are used in my study. The ability of patients to put these function words into the right position and to arrange the order of subject, object, and verb will be used to test the predictions of each model.

The paper is structured as follows. First of all, I will summarize the claims of each model. Then the unique properties of Chinese morphology and word order will be characterized. Based on these unique properties, each model makes different predictions. The experiment which is designed to test the predictions of the models will be elaborated, and the results and discussion presented. The data argue for the language-dominant model but also suggest a processing account for syndrome differences.

The Syndrome-Dominant Model

The syndrome-dominant model, which has been based primarily on data from English-speaking aphasics, classifies aphasia into subcategories according to syndrome. Among these types of aphasia, Broca's aphasia and Wernicke's aphasia are commonly recognized and known to occur across natural languages (Lesser 1978; Bates and Wulfeck 1989; Caramazza and Berndt 1978; Goodglass and Kaplan 1983).

Broca's aphasia is characterized by slow and halting speech, reduction of phrase length and syntactic complexity, disruption of normal prosody or melodic line, with a tendency to omit grammatical function words. Recently, the omission of closed class words has been claimed to be an essential property of Broca's aphasia (Berndt and Caramazza 1980; Caramazza and Berndt 1985; Goodglass and Kaplan 1983; Lesser 1978; Tissot, Mounin and Lhermitte 1973). It has also been reported that Broca's aphasics have agrammatic comprehension, parallel to their speech production (Bates et al. 1987; Bates and Wulfeck 1989; Bradley, Garret and Zurif 1980; Caramazza, Berndt, Basili and Koller 1981; Goodglass, Blumstein, Gleason, Hyde, Green and Statlender 1979; von Stockert and Bader 1976). This finding further suggests that Broca's aphasia reflects a central deficit of grammar (Berndt and Caramazza 1980; Bradley et al. 1980; Caramazza and Berndt 1985; Goodglass et al. 1979).

Wernicke's aphasia is characterized by fluent speech, with long sentences of considerable syntactic complexity. However, their expression is marked by severe word finding difficulties, circumlocution, and substitution of one word for another (Caramazza and Berndt 1978; Goodglass and Kaplan1983; Lesser 1978). These symptoms are attributed to a difficulty in retrieving open class word which is in contrast with closed class words.

The selective impairment of closed class words (i.e. Broca's aphasics) and that of open class word (i.e. Wernicke's aphasia) suggest that two word classes processed differently by the brain (Bradley 1978; Gordon and Caramazza 1983). This suggestion has universal implications which are worth studying with a non-inflected language, e.g. Chinese.

In the syndrome-dominant model, the violation of word order is not predicted to occur frequently in both Broca's and Wernicke's aphasics (Berndt and Caramazza 1980; Caramazza and Berndt 1985; Zurif and Grodzinsky 1983) although some studies have reported word order problems in Broca's aphasia (Saffran, Schwartz and Marin 1980; Schwartz, Saffran and Marin 1980). This finding suggests that Broca's aphasics basically have a central deficit of closed class words. By contrast, Wernicke's aphasics show a disruption of open class words.

The Language-Dominant Model

The major claim of the language-dominant model, which is based on cross-linguistic data is that variations in morphology and word order across languages indeed affect the symptoms of aphasics. There are languages with highly-inflected morphology, such as Italian, while there are languages without inflectional morphology, such as Chinese. Word order variation refers to the possible word orders in a language: for example, Italian allows greater word order variation than English does (MacWhinney, Bates and Kliegl 1984). The language-dominant model is supported by the finding that grammatical morphemes are crucial to sentence interpretation in highly-inflected languages. The finding is accounted for in terms of cue validity and cue cost.

Cue validity refers to the information value of a given grammatical, phonological or lexical cue to sentence meaning in a particular language. The information value is positively correlated with the frequency of the word, which means the "relative utility of words from the viewpoint of native speakers" (Bates 1988: 44). A morpheme is a valid cue when it is frequent and obligatory. For example, in Hungarian, the accusative marker is a valid cue for sentence interpretation because all object NPs are case-marked (MacWhinney and Osman-Sagy 1988). However, in English, only the first person and the third person pronouns are case-marked e.g. me, him, and them. The case marking system therefore is not a very powerful cue for English-speaking subjects in interpreting sentences. The language-dominant model predicts that aphasics will omit case marking when they are not valid cues but they will not omit case markings when they are very useful cues (Bates et al. 1987a).

However, valid cues may become invalid. For example, long-distance agreement, such as between subject and verb, which may not be adjacent, is much harder than a local case marker. This exception seems to revolve around aspects of cue cost. The notion of cue cost refers to the processing costs incurred in using a particular form-function mapping. Cue cost includes both the perceivability and assignability of the morpheme in question.

With respect to perceivability, perceptual difficulty may eliminate the validity of cues. For example, it is significantly harder to produce and perceive unstressed function words than stressed ones (Goodglass 1976; Kean 1979). Perceivability is also affected by frequency and semantic content of the morpheme (Bates and MacWhinney 1987; MacWhinney 1987a).

Assignability (e.g. of a closed class item to an open class one) is related to the memory demands placed on the sentence processor. Assignability has a big impact on closed class word (e.g. verbal suffixes) because most closed class words must be bound to a governing word or phrase. The ability to use closed class words therefore must include knowledge of both the governing content word and the closed class word. Thus, closed class words make a heavier demand on short term memory resources (Bates and MacWhinney 1987; MacWhinney 1987a). Assignability and perceivability constitute the notion of cue cost in the language-dominant model.

In regard to word order variations, it has been found that knowledge of ordering principles tends to be preserved in aphasia (Bates et al. 1988). These ordering principles include:

(1) the overuse of canonical word order by agrammatic patients when the language in question has a dominant word order; and
(2) the substitution of one word order for another when the language allows word order variations.

This claim of intact ordering is worth investigation because it suggests that agrammatic patients basically have a disruption of morphology rather than syntax.

The validity of morphological cues is different from one language to another since morphological cues in English and Chinese have different cue validity. The language-dominant model predicts a greater differentiation between Chinese Broca's aphasics and English Broca's aphasics and a lesser differentiation between Chinese Broca's aphasics and Chinese Wernicke's aphasics.

Morphology and Word Order in Mandarin Chinese

Chinese provides a unique opportunity to investigate these two models since there are very few closed class words but some word order variations in Chinese (Li and Thompson1981). The syndrome-dominant model therefore predicts that Chinese-speaking Broca's aphasics will suffer from a difficulty in closed class words while Chinese-speaking Wernicke's aphasics will be free from an impairment in closed class words. However, the language-dominant model predicts that both Broca's and Wernicke's aphasics will have difficulty with closed class words because these words cannot function as valid cues for Chinese-speakers in both speech comprehension and production.

Chinese is a non-inflected language. Concepts which are coded by closed class words in other languages, such as tense, number, semantic roles, are expressed by content words in Chinese. Aspect markers, the possessive marker, the adjective marker, the adverbial marker, and the relative clause marker are closed class words in Chinese but they co-exist with cognate content words. Appendix I illustrates Mandarin closed class words and their cognate content words (Chao 1968; Li and Thompson 1981; Wang 1946).

Among these function words, the aspectual markers, -le, -zhe, and -guo share similar syntactic , phonological, and semantic properties. Syntactically, the words -le, -zhe, and -guo serve as verbal suffixes forming sentence pattern like:

(1) subject + verb + -le + object
(2) subject + verb + -zhe + object
(3) subject + verb + -guo + object
(4) subject + verb + object + -le

These sentence patterns indicate that these words must follow the verb, except for -le in (4) which serves as a sentence final particle (Chao 1968; Li and Thompson 1981). Given these syntactic constraints, to be able to use

Chinese function words means that two necessary syntactic abilities are intact, i.e., the ability to build up a kernel sentence and to place a function word correctly. To test whether these abilities are preserved in Chinese aphasics, we investigate patients ability to place the three aspectual markers -le, -zhe, -guo. These morphemes consistently show up in the postverbal position. The form -le can also be a particle, which appears in sentence-final position; therefore -le is not a valid cue due to lack of consistent distribution. Moreover, all these aspectual markers are optional; they appear as verbal suffixes only when aspectual meaning is expressed in sentences. This optionality leads to the prediction that -le, -zhe, and -guo have relatively low cue validity in processing sentences. Among these three grammatical markers, -le is the least valid cue because it can appear in the verb-final and the sentence-final positions.

Etymologically, these three function words originally come from three cognate content words, liao, zhao, and guo. In modern Mandarin, function words and their cognate content words co-exist but these cognate words are used less frequently. Their phonological representations are:

Suffixes	Cognate Words	
-le	liao	"to complete"
-zhe	zhao	"to locate"
-guo	guo	"to pass"

The consonants of the words are the same as those found in the cognate words, but the vowels are neutralized into a schwa and the tones are atonic (neutralized). This neutralization of vowels and tones in function words implies that there is a phonological weakening process when cognate words change into function words. This weakening process suggests that neutral tones of these three function words should be regarded as phonologically unsalient.

As the phonological properties of function word weaken, their semantic functions also become reduced to aspect markers:

	Cognate Words	Suffixes
liao/-le	to complete	perfective aspect
zhao/-zhe	to locate	progressive aspect
guo/-guo	to pass	experiential aspect

Semantic opacity, together with phonological unsaliency, increases the cost of cues in language processing. The high cost of cues makes these function words difficult for native speakers to process.

Based on their syntactic, phonological, and semantic properties, the language-dominant model suggests that Chinese aphasics will show impairment in placing these function words.

In regard to word order, the syndrome-dominant model proposes that a violation of word order will not occur in aphasics' speech because an intact ability to use word order of English Broca's and Wernicke's aphasia has frequently been reported (Gleason, Goodglass, Green, Ackerman, and Hyde 1975; Ansell and Flower 1982; Bates et al. 1987a; Bates et al. 1988). By contrast, the language-dominant model suggests that a misuse of word order can happen in languages with word order variation e.g. Italian (Bates et al. 1987a; Bates et al. 1988).

According to Li and Thompson (1981), the basic word order for Mandarin is SVO for sentences that have subjects and objects. However, there are word order variations. An object can be topicalized or passivized to make an OSV sentence, the disposal marker -BA can be inserted into sentences to make SOV sentence. A VOS sentence can occur in relative clauses. Of these six possible word order variations, OVS and VSO are impossible in Mandarin Chinese.

Given the morphological properties and word order variations in Chinese, the prediction made by the syndrome dominant model is that Chinese Broca's aphasics will demonstrate a significant impairment in closed class words while Wernicke's aphasics will be free from the impairment. Both types of aphasics should show no significant error in the domi-

Table 1. Various Word Orders of Mandarin Chinese

Word order	Examples
SVO	I eat (le) rice (le). I have eaten the rice.
SOV	I, rice eat (le). This is I who ate the rice.
OSV	Rice, I eat (le). This is the rice that I ate.
VOS	Eat rice (de) I. (This is a relative clause) I who ate the rice.
*OVS	Rice eat I I eat rice.
*VSO	eat I rice I eat rice.

nant word order. On the other hand, the language-dominant model predicts that both Broca's and Wernicke's aphasics will suffer from a deficit in closed class words because closed class words are not valid cues in Chinese. Patients may show word order variation within the normal range because there are word order variations in Chinese.

Experiment 1 Sentence Arrangement Subjects

In this experiment, nine Broca's aphasics, six Wernicke's aphasics, and six control subjects were asked to arrange cards depicting Chinese characters in sequence.[1] These aphasics have been screened by speech therapists in Taiwan. A modified version of Boston Diagnostic Aphasic Exam (BDAE) provided criteria for aphasic classification. Among nine Broca's aphasics, there are four moderate cases and five severe cases. The six Wernicke's aphasics included three severe cases and three mild cases. Controls were selected by matching the age, sex, and birth place with those of aphasics. The history of the subjects is summarized in Table 2. (More detailed information is reported in Appendix 2)

Materials

In this experiment, two sets of sentence patterns were used. Each set consisted of eight randomized sentences. Each sentence included one pronoun (ta), one verb, one function word, and one noun. These words are monosyllabic (single character); characters were written on square paper boards (2cm x 2cm). In testing, the four characters used in each sentence were set in a simple grid, for example,

hua (flower)	zhe (-ing)
ta (he)	jiao (water)

Procedure

Before testing began, the experimenter showed the subjects the four characters to be used.[2] The subjects were required to identify these four

Table 2. History of Subjects

	Broca's	*Wernicke's*	*Controls*
Number	9	6	6
Mean of Age	50	47	47
Education	13	8	13
Post-Onset	12 yrs-6 ms	2 yrs-3 ms	*

characters, and then arranged them into a sentence. The subjects were first informed that these characters could be arranged into a sentence. If a subject did not seem to understand the task or refused to participate, the demonstrator showed him/her how to proceed. Since the four characters used were arranged in simple grid-like fashion, with two placed in the top box and two in the bottom ones, the experimenter was able to rotate the position of these characters during the experiment. The subjects relied upon the traditional style of Chinese writing and, hence, arranged their words vertically. If subjects showed any uncertainty as to how their words should be arranged, the demonstrator noted it on the answer sheet, urging them to undertake the task.

Analysis

In analyzing the data thus collected. we direct our attention toward trying to discern:

(1) whether the position of function words chosen by Broca's aphasics was similar to Wernicke's aphasics and control subjects.
(2) whether SVO word order was relatively intact in both Broca's aphasics and Wernicke's aphasics.
(3) whether individual differences within an aphasic group was similar to the differences between groups, with respect to (1) and (2).

Results and Discussion

The results in Table 3 indicate that Broca's aphasics used (96%) correct SVO word order which is better than Wernicke's aphasics (69%) in producing the order of subject, verb and object. However, Broca's aphasics put the function word in the correct position (with only 37% correct function

Table 3. The Percentage of Correct SVO Word Order and Correct Verb-Function Word Order

	SVO	F-word
Broca's	.96 (.93)	.37 (.27)
Wernicke's	.69 (.39)	.69 (.39)
Controls	1.0	1.0

The data in parentheses indicate the responses of the four severely impaired Broca's aphasics and three severely impaired Wernicke's aphasics.

Table 4. The Distribution of Subject on SVO Word Order and V-Suffix

No. of SVO		No. of subject	
	Broca's	Wernicke's	Controls
6	7	3	6
5	2		
4		1	
3			
2		1	
1		1	
0			

		No. of subject	
No. of F-words	Broca's	Wernicke's	Controls
6		3	6
5			
4	1	1	
3	3		
2	4	1	
1		1	
0	1		

word) less frequently than Wernicke's aphasics (with 69% correct function word). Thus, the results at first appear to support the syndrome dominant model, which claims that Broca's aphasics are impaired in function words while Wernicke's aphasics are free from a disruption of function words.

However, the data of severely impaired Broca's and Wernicke's aphasics show that their ability to arrange SVO word order is significantly different (93% vs. 39% respectively) while their ability to put function words in the correct position is only slightly different (27% vs. 39% respectively). This finding suggests that both Chinese Broca's aphasics and Wernicke's aphasics are impaired in closed class words. These findings motivate a detailed analysis of individual responses in the sentence arranging task.

In Table 4, a detailed analysis of individual responses in arranging sentences shows that there is insufficient evidence to support the syndrome-dominant model. With respect to correct placement of function words, an overlap is found between severe Broca's aphasics and severe Wernicke's aphasics. This finding cannot be accounted for by the syndrome-dominant model, which claims that Broca's aphasics are impaired in closed class words, and Wernicke's aphasics are impaired in open class words. Instead, we must appeal to the language-dominant model in order to account for the similar performance of severe Broca's aphasics and severe Wernicke's aphasics. Both severe Broca's aphasics and severe Wernicke's aphasics are unable to put function words in the right position when these words do not serve as a sufficient cue in language processing.

Table 5. Word Order Variation

Controls					
	ta	he	cha	36/36	
	he	drink	tea		
Broca's aphasics					
	ta	he	cha	(SVO)	53/56
	he	drink	tea		
	ta	cha	he	(SOV)	1/56
	he	tea	drink		
	cha	ta	he	(OSV)	1/56
	tea	he	drink		
	*he	ta	cha	(VSO)	1/56
	drink	he	tea		
Wernicke's aphasics					
	ta	jian	zhi	(SVO)	25/36
	he	cut	paper		
	ta	zhi	jian	(SOV)	4/36
	he	paper	cut		
	xi	shou	ta	(VOS)	5/36
	wash	hand	he		
	*xi	ta	wan	(VSO)	1/36
	wash	he	bowl		
	*yan	chou	ta	(OVS)	1/36
	cigar	smoke	he		

Moreover, another finding, namely, that Broca's aphasics strongly prefer SVO word order but Wernicke's aphasics show great word order variation, manifests syndrome differences. In Table 5, the results show that the Wernicke's aphasics use a wider range of order variation than the Broca's aphasics and most of variations fall into the normal range of variation. Broca's aphasics have less variation, while controls always use SVO word order. These findings suggest that word order variation but not the open-closed class word distinction can account for the difference Chinese-speaking Broca's aphasics and Wernicke's aphasics.

Conclusion

To summarize, this study shows that

(1) both Broca's aphasics and Wernicke's aphasics are impaired in the placement of function words. The problem of both severely impaired Broca's aphasics and Wernicke's aphasics reflect the paucity of morphology in Chinese.

(2) Wernicke's aphasics show a greater variation of word order than Broca's aphasics. Interestingly, most of order patterns reflect possible word orders in Chinese.

These data argue for the language-dominant model, which claims that Broca's aphasics rely on canonical word order as a "safe harbor" when their native language has a dominant word order (e.g. SVO in Chinese), in contrast, Wernicke's aphasics show a wide range of word order variation due to their lexical selection problems (Bates et al. 1988; Bates et al., 1989). Thus, the present findings on impairment in closed class words support the two basic claims of the language-dominant model (Bates et al. 1987; Bates et al. 1988; Bates et al. 1989; MacWhinney et al. 1984)

(1) Morphology is vulnerable in all types of aphasia.

(2) Morphological differences between languages affect aphasic symptoms.

Notes

*I would like to acknowledge the valuable suggestions given to me by Professor Elizabeth Bates and Professor Ovid Tzeng in the preparation of the paper. I would also like to thank Professor Patricia Clancy and Professor Elaine Andersen for their helpful comments on this paper. This research is based on a master thesis by the author completed at Fu-Jen Catholic University in Taiwan, in 1984, under the direction of professor Shuang-fan Huang.

1. The sentence arrangement is designed to examine patients' ability ot use word order and closed class words and to eliminate the affect of non-linguistic impairments, such as the memory span deficit and the motor speech disorder, on patients' performance. This task is not a metalinguistic task because, instead of forcing subjects to judge the grammaticality of sentences, we allow subjects to freely make sentences with given four words.

2. Before arranging sentences, subjects have to pass a sentence comprehension test, which is similar to the sentence arrangement task concerning the length and the content of sentences.

References

Ansell, B. and C. Flowers. 1982. "Aphasic Adults' Use of Heuristic and Structural Linguistic Cues for Analysis". *Brain and Language* 16.61-72.

Bates, E. 1988. *Cross-linguistic Studies: The Annual Report*. up.

Bates, E., A.D. Friederici and B. Wulfeck. 1987a. "Comprehension in Aphasia: A cross-linguistic Study". *Brain and Language* 32.19-67.

Bates, E., A.D. Friederici, and B. Wulfeck. 1987b. "Grammatical Morphology in Aphasia: Evidence from Three Languages". *Cortex* 23.545-547.

Bates, E., A.D. Friederici, B. Wulfeck and L. Juarez. 1988. "On the Preservation of Word Order in Aphasia: Cross-linguistic Evidence". *Brain and Language* 33.323-346.

Bates, E. and B. MacWhinney. 1987. "Competition, Variation and Language Learning". MacWhinney 1987.157-193.

Bates, E. and B. Wulfeck. 1989. *Cross-linguistic Study of Sentence Processing*. Cambridge: Cambridge Univ. Press.

Berndt, R.S. and A. Caramazza. 1980. "A Redefinition of the Syndrome of Broca's Aphasia: Implications for a Neuropsychological Model of Language". *Applied Psycholinguistics* 1.225-278.

Bradley, D.C. 1978. *Computational Distinction of Verbal Types*. Doctoral dissertation. Massachusetts Institute of Technology.

Bradley, D.C., M.F. Garret and E.B. Zurif. 1980. "Syntactic Deficits in Broca's Aphasia". *Biological Studies of Mental Processes* ed. by D. Caplan. Cambridge, MA: MIT Press.

Caramazza, A. and R.S. Berndt. 1978. "Semantic and Syntactic Processes in Aphasia: A Review of the Literature". *Psychological Bulletin* 85.898-918.

Caramazza, A. and R.S. Berndt. 1985. "A Multi-component Deficit View of Agrammatic Broca's Aphasia". Kean 1985.

Caramazza, A., R.S. Berndt, A.G. Basili, and J.J. Koller. 1981. "Syntactic Processing Deficits in Aphasia". *Cortex* 17.333-348.

Caramazza, A. and E.B. Zurif. 1976. "Dissociation of Algorithmic and Heuristic Processes in Language Comprehension: Evidence from aphasia". *Brain and Language* 3.572-582.

Chao. 1968. *A Grammar of Spoken Chinese*. Berkeley and Los Angeles: University of California Press.

Chen, S. 1984. *An Investigation of Chinese Aphasics: With Special Reference to Four Function Words*. MA Thesis. Taiwan: Fu-Jen Catholic University.

Chen, S. and J. Wu. 1985. "The Boston Diagnostic Aphasic Exam: A Modified Version in Chinese". ms.

Gleason, J.B., H. Goodglass, E. Green, N. Ackerman, and H.R. Hyde. 1975. "The Retrieval of Syntax in Broca's Aphasia". *Brain and Language* 2.451-471.

Goodglass, H., 1976. "Agrammatism". *Studies on Neurolinguistics. Vol. 1* ed. by H. Whitaker and H.A. Whitaker. New York: Academic Press.

Goodglass, H., S.E. Blumstein, J.B. Gleason, M.R. Hyde, E. Green and S. Statlender. 1979. "The Effect of Syntactic Encoding on Sentence Comprehension in Aphasia". *Brain and Language* 7.201-209.

Goodglass, H. and E. Kaplan. 1983. *The Assessment of Aphasia and Related DIsorders (2nd ed)*. Philadelphia: Lea & Febiger.

Goodglass, H. and L. Menn. 1985. "Is Agrammatism a Unitary Phenomenon?" Kean 1985.

Gordon, B. and A. Caramazza. 1983. "Closed and Open Class Lexical Access in Agrammatic and Fluent Aphasics". *Brain and Language* 16.335-345.

Kean, M.L. 1979. "Agrammatism: A Phonological Deficit?" *Cognition* 7.69-84.

Kean, M.L., ed. 1985. *Agrammatism*. New York: Academic Press.

Lesser, R. 1978. *Linguistic Investigation of Aphasia. London: Edward Arnold.*

Li, C. and S.A. Thompson. 1981. *Mandarin Chinese: A Functional Reference Grammar*. Berkeley: University of California Press.

MacWhinney, B. 1987. "The Competition Model". MacWhinney 1987.249-308.

MacWhinney, B, ed. 1987. *Mechanism of Language Acquisition*. Hillsdale, NJ: Erlbaum.

MacWhinney, B., E. Bates and R. Kliegl. 1984. "Cue Validity and Sentence Interpretation in English, German, and Italian". *Journal of Verbal Learning and Verbal Behavior* 23.127-150.

MacWhinney, B. and J. Osman-Sagy. 1988. "Grammatical Impairments in Hungarian. Paper presented in Academy of Aphasia, Montreal.

Saffran, E.M., M.F. Schwartz and O.S.M. Marin. 1980. "The Word Order Problem in Agrammatism II: Production." *Brain and Language* 10.263-280.

Schwartz, M.F., E. Saffran, and O.S.M. Marin. 1980. The Word Order Problem in Agrammatism I: Comprehension". *Brain and Language* 10.249-262.

Slobin, D., and A. Talay. 1988. "Grammatical Impairments in Turkish". Paper presented in Academy of Aphasia, Montreal.

Smith, S., and E. Bates. 1987. "Accessibility of Case and Gender Contrasts for Assignment of Agent-object Relations in Broca's Aphasics and Fluent Anomics. *Brain and Language* 30.8-32.

Smith, S. and L. Mimica. 1984. "Agrammatism in a Case-infected Language". *Brain and Language* 13.274-290.

Tzeng, O.Z.L., and S. Chen. 1988. "Grammatical Impairments in Chinese". Paper Presented in Academy of Aphasia, Montreal.

Tissot, R.J., G. Mounin and F. Lhermitte. 1973. *L'Agrammatisme*. Brussel: Dessart.

von Stockert, T.R. and L. Bader. 1976. "Some Relations of Grammar and Lexicon in Aphasia". *Cortex* 12.49-60.

Wang, L. 1946. *Hanyu Shigao* (The History of The Chinese Language). Shanghai: The Commercial Printing House.

Zurif, E.B. and Y. Grodzinsky. 1983. "Sensitivity to Grammatical Structure in Agrammatic Aphasics: A Reply to Linebarger, Schwartz, and Saffran". *Cognition* 15.

Appendix 1

Mandarin Closed Class Words

	Function Words	*Content Words*
Tense	*	today, yesterday...
plural	-men	some, several, many
Gender	*	nouns such as women, men...
Aspect	-le -zhe -guo zai-	These aspectual markers co-exist with their cognate content words which bear stressed.
Agreement	classifiers	*
Possession	-de	It coexists with its cognate content word which bears stressed.
Adj marker	-de	
Adv marker	-de	
Relative-Clause marker	-de	
Semantic roles	prepositions which are also verbs	nominal localizer such as inside, outside, top-side usually go with coverb 'to locate'
Pronouns	pronouns	

Appendix 2

History of Subjects

	Age	Sex	Education	Post-Onset	Etiology	Lesion
Broca's						
#1 CMM	58	F	16 yrs	12 yrs	CVA	F-T-P
#2 CSY	63	M	16 yrs	12 months	CVA	(hemiplegia)
#3 YJQ	28	M	12 yrs	3 yrs	Head injury	F-T-P
#4 ZJN	40	M	12 yrs	6 months	Hemor	F-T-P
#5 WDS	45	M	12 yrs	6 months	Hemor	F-P
#6 LDY	46	M	11 yrs	15 months	CVA	F-T-P
#7 HY	60	M	9 yrs	6 months	Hemor	F-P
#8 ZZZ	53	M	12 yrs	4 yrs	CVA	F-T-P-O
#9 LST	55	M	16 yrs	6 months	Hemor	F-T
Wernicke's						
#10 LWZ	33	F	12 yrs	3 months	Hemor	T-P
#11 LZL	45	M	6 yrs	3 months	Tumor	T-P
#12 ZJY	65	M	9 yrs	6 months	CVA	T-P-O
#13 FZS	61	M	6 yrs	4 months	CVA	T-P
#14 LWJ	13	F	6 yrs	3 months	Head injury	
T#15 LYT	66	M	9 yrs	2 yrs	CVA	T-P-O
Controls						
#16	43	M	8 yrs	*	*	*
#17	55	F	14 yrs	*	*	*
#18	61	M	16 yrs	*	*	*
#19	30	M	12 yrs	*	*	*
#20	37	M	12 yrs	*	*	*
#21	56	M	16 yrs	*	*	*

Speech Pathology and SLA

Synergy in Applied Linguistics:

Theoretical and Pedagogical Implications

Jack S. Damico
The University of Southwestern Louisiana

Individuals surveying the applied linguistic fields of teaching English as a second language (ESL) and speech-language pathology will note striking similarities between these two disciplines. They mirror one another in their evolution: they began with similar objectives, were side-tracked from those objectives by their utilization of a powerful theoretical construct and have recently moved toward a re-establishment of their original missions. Specifically, these disciplines were influenced early in their development by empiricism and an autonomous conception of language that turned them away from functional considerations and toward a structural focus that influenced both testing and teaching applications. For an extensive period of time, therefore, there was a lack of appreciation for an integrative or interactive construct of language upon which to base pedagogy.

This state of affairs has changed over the past two decades, however, and there has been a discernible shift in both of these disciplines toward a synergistic conception of language. That is, the theoretical constructs utilized in conducting research and guiding pedagogical practice are beginning to stress the interactions between the traditionally defined levels or components of language (e.g., morphology, syntax, phonology) and between language and other intrinsic systems like memory and intelligence. Further, the influence of numerous variables extraneous to the language learner are now being incorporated into theories of language acquisition. This has resulted in a much more dynamic and functional conception of language. At least on a practical level, these fields are rejecting traditional assessment and pedagogical approaches and are moving toward more "interactive", "naturalistic" and "socially valid" approaches.

It is interesting to note, however, that although these fields seem to exhibit parallel development, this movement toward synergy has been undertaken with a different focus in these two disciplines due to different foundational beliefs. The results of this separate but parallel evolution is that each field has developed unique but relevant data which can be of value to the other. It is the objective of this paper to discuss some of the ways that professionals involved in teaching English as a second language and those functioning as speech-language pathologists can increase their interactions with one another for their mutual benefit. Such interaction will lead to a second type of synergy — a professional variety. That is, the results of the interactions between these two disciplines will be greater than what could be predicted by looking at either discipline considered separately. A brief review of the evolution of these two applied linguistic fields and a discussion of recent theoretical and empirical work will clarify their similarities and differences and reveal how each discipline may benefit from the other.

Parallels Within a Historical Perspective

Discussions of the development of both ESL and speech-language pathology indicate that these two fields have undergone three distinct changes during the last sixty years and are rapidly completing a fourth modification. With some variation, these changes across the two fields are quite similar. A review of each can easily demonstrate these similarities.

Teaching English as a Second Language

In his review of second language teaching and testing issues, Bernard Spolsky (1978) suggested that there were three clearly divisible periods in the evolution of teaching English as a second language. Until the 1930s, ESL functioned in what Spolsky referred to as the "pre-scientific period". During this period, language teachers held an overriding interest in functional considerations. They were concerned with student performance and success in terms of the effectiveness of language use outside of the classroom and little emphasis was placed on theoretical foundations and statistical validation. The major pedagogical guides to classroom practices and evaluation were the judgement of the experienced teacher and social validation. Consequently, the focus was on providing speakers with the skills to use language effectively. Even as early as the 1830s, pattern drills and grammar exercises which separated classroom activity from actual communication were argued against in the literature (Drake 1977).

During the 1930s, however, the social sciences in the United States were heavily influenced by the doctrine of empiricism and teaching English as a second language was no exception. Through the influence of Leonard Bloomfield (1933; 1939) and his colleagues (Weiss, 1925), American linguistics — and by extension teaching English as a second language — became heavily influenced by behaviorism. A strict empiricist, Bloomfield believed that the only data to consider in the study of language was that which was directly observable. He stated that the relationship between the corpus of data and the theoretical description of language had to be a direct one. He also believed that general linguistics was more a body of techniques of description to accommodate this objective than it was a body of beliefs about the nature of language. Structural description rather than explanation became the objective of linguistics. As Fred Newmeyer (1980) described it, linguistic description was a,

> catalogue of observables and statements in principle extracted directly from observables by a set of mechanical procedures. (p. 5)

Based on this taxonomic perspective of the American structuralists, ESL entered what Spolsky referred to as the "psychometric-structuralist period" which continued from the early 1930s until the early 1960s. During this period, language and other human abilities were viewed as conglomerations of many distinguishable elements each pertaining to some distinct domain or component. Language proficiency was viewed as consisting of separable components of phonology, morphology, lexicon, syntax, and so on, each which could be further divided into distinct inventories of elements (i.e., sounds, classes of sounds or phonemes, syllables, morphemes, words, idioms, phrase structures). This conception of language proficiency led to a focus on the structural aspects of language and away from the earlier emphasis on functionality of communication. Further, the autonomy of language from other abilities and the reduction of language proficiency into components and smaller items resulted in a movement away from the interaction of language with its contextual variables and even the integration of language levels with one another. The result was that the naive synergy of the pre-scientific period was eliminated.

During this psychometric-structuralist period the most enthusiastic proponents of this view argued that during evaluations each test item should focus on only one element of one component at a time (Fries 1952; Lado 1961). It was urged that items testing phonemic contrasts should not be mixed with those aimed at testing vocabulary knowledge which should, in turn, be distinguished from items aimed at syntactic patterns and so forth. It was further argued that a test could not be valid if it mixed several skills or levels of language structure (Lado 1961). In this period, presumably the ideal assessment would involve the evaluation of each of the domains of structure and each of the skills of interest and then all the results could be combined to form a total picture of language proficiency.

The approach to language pedagogy, of course, mirrored this approach to assessment. It was considered scientific and innovative to teach discrete language elements, patterns, or items in some predetermined sequence. This was usually accomplished through pattern drills or exercises stressing maximal exposure and repetitive practice with the target structures rather than the earlier focus on language as communication.

This psychometric-structuralist period, however, came under increasing criticism in the 1960s. In 1961, for example, John B. Carroll commented on the artificial character of the discrete point approach which was generated during this period. He stated that it was impossible in principle to devise fully discrete items in real testing situations or in teaching environments. A major problem with these discrete point approaches was that they did not take into account the necessity of the context during language learning or use. Compensating for these weaknesses, Carroll referred to another kind of test and pedagogical approach — one aimed at more global properties of language ability. He termed this the "integrative approach". Carroll's critique of the discrete point methodology that dominated the psychometric-structuralist period and his suggestion for a more integrative and less autonomous approach to language testing and teaching was indicative of the next developmental stage.

This "integrative-sociolinguistic period" tended to re-focus attention in ESL on the synergistic quality of language. This period, extending from the 1960s until early in the 1980s, was characterized by the way that language proficiency was conceptualized. Language proficiency was viewed as a composite construct with holistic qualities that was best assessed and taught within the rich context of discourse. This view of language proficiency stimulated the formulation of a construct of language proficiency that was diametrically opposed to the autonomous and discrete point conception of language advocated in the previous historical period. Known as the "Unitary Factor Hypothesis", this conception stated that language proficiency might not be decomposable at all and that it could be assessed with nearly equal validity in a great variety of ways. All that was necessary was that language be allowed to function integratively (Oller, 1979).

Just as with the extreme view that language was completely autonomous and divisible into numerous components, however, the unitary hypothesis which stressed no divisibility was equally extreme and invalid. Research soon established that language proficiency is componentially complex (Bachman and Palmer 1983; Carroll 1983; Upshur and Homburg 1983) and the theories of language proficiency moved more to the center of the divisibility-unitary continuum. This was because less extreme variations of integrative theory had some validity. While the items of discrete point tests were designed to focus on one single element of one component of grammar removed from contextual variables, integrative tests required the use of many elements across several linguistic levels embedded in contextual variables — and all these items interacted simultaneously. This approach was more consistent with the synergistic quality of language and yielded more valid measurements of language proficiency (Oller 1973; Spolsky 1968; Upshur 1967; Valette 1964). Second language testing researchers embraced this approach.

In general, a similar advantage was noted for the more integrative and contextually embedded approach over the autonomous and artificial methods in language pedagogy. There was a call for less reliance on the drill and skill routines of the psychometric-structuralist period and more reliance on the functional and/or notional approaches both in terms of pedagogical activities and syllabi design (Brown and Yule 1983; Oller and Richard-Amato 1983; Wilkins 1976). Additionally, more interactive and meaning-based pedagogical methods were advocated (e.g., the Natural Approach, Community Language Learning, Total Physical Response).

Most unique to the ESL field during the integrative- sociolinguistic period, however, was the increased interest in potential learning variables extraneous to language ability itself. Numerous researchers recognized the wide variation common to the language learning situation and realized that other variables needed to be considered. Specifically, non-linguistic factors were incorporated into the synergistic equation advocated during the integrative-sociolinguistic period.

Three general types of non-linguistic variables were investigated during this period: affective learner variables, sociological variables, and access variables. The affective variables primarily involved issues regarding motivation, learner attitudes, risk taking, and anxiety. For example, Gardner and Lambert (1972) conducted numerous studies on the role of motivation in second language acquisition. The two types of motivation they identified — integrative and instrumental — were based on what the learner hoped to achieve by learning a second language. They found that motivational differences significantly impacted on a learner's success in acquiring a second language. Another affective variable of interest that was researched was learner attitudes toward the target language.

Numerous studies (Gardner 1985) indicated that learner attitudes could have an effect. One clear illustration of just such an effect was reported by John Schumann in his 1978 case study of a Spanish-speaking immigrant who held negative attitudes about English. Due to his attitude, this individual restricted his language exposure opportunities and consistently favored his first language. As a result, this apparently normal language learner fossilized in his acquisition of English at a very rudimentary level. Finally, learner anxiety or even the willingness to take risks and make mistakes during second language learning has been investigated under the concept of "ego permeability" (Guiora 1972).

Regarding sociological factors, ESL researchers have studied listener reaction, the effects of negative attitudes toward the learner's first language and home culture, error gravity, and the effects that maximal versus minimal exposure and opportunities may have. The data indicate that each factor plays an important role in second language learning (Klein 1986). One area of investigation is particularly interesting given the movement toward functionism. These studies investigated the error gravity of certain types of errors. That is, the effects that particular types of errors have on communication. Error gravity was investigated in two ways. First, the direct effect of production errors was noted by focusing on the degree to which the errors affect comprehensibility in listeners. Johansson (1975) found that although all errors were generally noticed, errors of pronunciation, morphology, tone and surface level syntax did not impede comprehensibility. Albrechtsen and colleagues (1979) found that errors of discourse were far more impeding on communication than were structural problems. The only exception were significant problems with semantics.

The second type of error gravity — indirect effect — has also been investigated. These investigations focused on the ways teachers and others reacted to errors in the classroom. Fanselow (1977) found that teachers reacted more to errors of meaning than to grammatical errors. Similarly, Burton and Samuda (1980) found that students typically react and express the need for additional information only on each other's errors of communicative intent rather than on grammatical correctness.

The third general set of non-linguistic factors investigated by researchers during the integrative-sociolinguistic period were the effects that access variables have on the language learning process. Numerous studies have focused on the difference between "learning versus acquisition" (Krashen 1981), "guided versus spontaneous learning" (Corder 1973), "formal versus informal" learning or "artificial versus naturalistic" opportunities (Upshur and Palmer 1974; Palmer 1978). Other access variables included the quality of language input received by the language learner (Ferguson 1977; Ferguson and de Bose 1977), the teaching methods used, and the exposure time needed for learning to occur.

These studies are illustrations of the manner with which ESL has addressed the synergistic quality of language by figuring non-linguistic factors into the language learning equation. The primary point, of course, is that these studies are indicative of the movement back to more synergy in language and toward a more naturalistic and functional perspective.

Speech-Language Pathology

A review of the field of speech-language pathology from a historical perspective does reveal similarities. This discipline also began from a functional perspective and initially focused on effectiveness in communication. Woobert in his 1920 article, "Pathological conditions, speech defects", stressed the functional disadvantages and the impact that poor speech had on a speaker's self-concept. Similarly, Lee Edward Travis and the first graduates in the profession (from the University of Iowa program) stressed the need to make speakers effective communicators despite their difficulties. The focus during the beginnings of speech-language pathology as a profession was clearly functional and it paralleled ESL's pre-scientific period.

Due to the influence of psychology on the beginning of speech-language pathology as a profession, however, this functional orientation shifted. As Watson's emphasis on behaviorism became dominant in American psychology and thereby influenced the area of intelligence testing and psychometrics, this focus on rigid psychometric design was embraced in speech-language pathology from the 1930s until the 1970s. The most significant early attempts to adopt this rigid psychometric approach to language assessment and treatment in speech-language pathology came from Lee Edward Travis (Travis and Rasmus 1931) and Samuel Robbins (1933). This fact in itself was important. These two men were perhaps the most influential in the fledgling profession. Travis was the first Ph.D. in the field of speech correction and is considered by many to be the "Father of the Profession". Robbins, a professor of psychology at Emerson College, was very well known. He served as the President of the American Speech Correction Association twice in the early years and also served as the organization's first permanent secretary. The fact that these two men preferred the more rigid psychometric approach to the earlier focus on functionality undoubtedly had an impact on the field. The study and treatment of language and communication disorders became more "scientific".

In the mid 1950s this psychometric emphasis was joined in speech-language pathology by the structural linguistic methodologies that so influenced ESL. The first article in the speech and language literature that stressed the value of structural linguistics was written by M.H. Scargill (1954). This paper, "Modern linguistics and recovery from aphasia" encouraged the application of structural linguistic methodology to the study of clinical populations. Citing the work of Fries (1952), Scargill made an appeal to language correctionists to take advantage of this advanced social science.

This approach to description was exactly what the language correctionists desired. The branches of linguistic description that were focused upon by the descriptivists — phonology, morphology and syntax — were easily observable and could be placed into a psychometric framework. Additionally, the descriptivist constraint against level mixing and the rejection of meaning as a valid target of analysis (Bloomfield 1933) allowed for a theoretical defense of highly artificial but standardized tests.

Within several years, the influence of structural linguistics was easily recognized in the area of language assessment. The 1957 American Speech and Hearing Association Convention provided a sectional meeting entitled, "Speech from the viewpoint of linguistic science", and authors like Strauss and McCarus (1958) suggested incorporating structural linguistic techniques into the assessment of clinical populations. Some professionals were even more adamant about this new input source. C.K. Thomas (1957), for example, in a review of Henry L. Smith Jr.'s Linguistic Science and the Teaching of English stated,

> Speech and Hearing Clinics and Departments of Speech can no more ignore basic linguistics than physicians and surgeons can ignore basic anatomy and physiology. (p. 398)

By far the most impressive indicator of the structural linguistic input, however, were the tests and therapy techniques developed during this time period and their explicit or implicit reliance on the descriptivist techniques. One test in particular deserves special comment. In reporting some of the experimental data on his Michigan Picture Language Inventory — the first standardized structural language tool in speech-language pathology — Lerea (1958) indicated that this tool was based upon the work of Charles Fries (1952). He selected the work of Fries because it allowed him to use vocabulary and syntax which were readily amenable to the rigors of psychometric design and standardization. Lerea recommended this type of approach for all test designers and stressed the importance of the American structuralist input. With the work of Lerea, the field of language assessment saw the first application of the more rigid and demanding psychometric criteria recognized by the APA and its integration with this dominant school of American linguistics. The linguistic connection was now firmly established.

This development in the evolution of speech-language pathology, of course, closely parallels that described earlier as the psychometric-structural period in teaching English as a second language. Both began in the 1930s and both stressed the autonomy of language and embraced the discrete point methodology. Whereas ESL entered a new period around the early 1960s, however, speech-language pathology remained heavily influenced by this methodology until the mid-1970s. For the most part, the tests designed (e.g., the Berry-Talbott Exploratory Test of Grammar; the Test for Auditory Comprehension of Language; Assessment of Children's Language Comprehension; Northwestern Syntax Screening Test) and the therapy techniques utilized (e.g., Developmental Syntax Program; Teaching American Language to Kids; Folkes Sentence Building) stressed all the qualities of the psychometric-structuralist period.

In the mid-1970s, however, changes were occurring. There was a movement toward more naturalistic assessment and a growing focus on functional components. There were various reasons for this change. First, several clinical reports or case studies had been reported in the literature in the latter part of the 1960s which suggested that there were problems with the heavy reliance on the autonomous and discrete point conception of language. Lieberman (1965) reported on a child who wouldn't ask for a repetition when one was needed for comprehension. The child had definite language problems but the language tests were too focused on structural and artificial tasks to be able to identify such a functional problem. Other case studies followed. Rosenberg (1966) called the validity of the current approach into question, Paul Weiner (1967) and Monsees and Berman (1968) questioned the effectiveness of the psychometric-structural approach in terms of the underlying constructs, and Blue (1975) demonstrated that the psychometric tests were not effective in identifying children who were "marginal communicators".

The second influence was more research oriented. In 1969, Shriner, Holloway, and Daniloff presented data that questioned the appropriateness of considering phonological deficits as independent from other aspects of linguistic behavior. Shriner stressed the possibility of a synergy of linguistic disorders. In rapid succession, John Panagos (1974) and others published empirical data which supported Shriner's postulation. This work moved speech-language pathology toward a more integrative conception of language.

Finally, several researchers were modifying the discrete point approach to language assessment and suggesting the utilization of context in a manner similar to those efforts made by John B. Carroll in ESL several years earlier. Siegel in 1967, Laura Lee and Gerald Canter in 1971, and Leonard (1972), Tyack (1972) and Streng (1972) all advocated a more contextually appropriate set of procedures for data collection and analysis.

The movement toward greater functional considerations and synergy in the manner seen in ESL was primarily established in speech-language pathology in the mid-1970s. John Muma (1975) published an article titled, "The communication game: Dump and play" which focused on the functionality of language. Soon after, Rees and Shulman (1978), Prutting (1979) and others advocated greater attention to the synergistic qualities of language and stressed the need for more functional applications. Gene Abkarian (1977) explicitly discussed the trend toward synergy in speech-language pathology in his article, "The changing face of a discipline: Isn't it romantic?" and Norma Rees (1979) utilized the theme of movement toward synergy in speech-language pathology in her 1979 Presidential address at the American Speech-Language-Hearing Association convention. Clearly, the field of speech-language pathology had re-established the earlier emphasis on synergy and functionality and this movement is apparent in the work conducted and published throughout the 1980s.

Although its development shadowed the evolution toward synergy in ESL by about 15 years, speech-language pathology's development in this direction is quite similar. The purpose of this historical review was to demonstrate that point.

A close consideration of this review, however, reveals more than just a striking similarity. There were also significant differences in the way that these two fields moved toward their current commonality. These differences are discussed in the next section.

Differences in the Movement to Synergy

Both ESL and speech-language pathology are currently at the stage where language is considered complex and synergistic. At least in practice, the artificial constraints of the autonomous conception of language are less evident in both of these fields of applied linguistics. Each of these disciplines, however, appear to have focused on different aspects of language synergy during their development. In doing so, each has established a wealth of empirical data, practical application, and theoretical insight which can complement the work of the other field. Consequently, these differences warrant further discussion.

ESL, a field which has been concerned with normal learners, has traditionally assumed that the language and/or learning faculties of these students or language users are adequate. Klein (1986), Krashen (1982), Spolsky (1988), Schumann (1978) and others routinely make this assumption. This belief had direct implications in ESL's movement toward synergy. Rather than focusing on the synergistic implications of language learning within the learner, ESL focused on extraneous factors. Hence the heavy emphasis on affective (non-faculty) variables, sociological variables, and access variables.

The field of speech-language pathology, however, was founded on an emphasis toward the individual learner and the absence of a normal or adequate language faculty. Due to the influence of the medical model, this profession assumed that performance differences were due primarily to intrinsic factors rather than extrinsic ones. Attention, therefore, has primarily been directed toward the individual and that learner's intrinsic system. This is the reason that case studies had the effects that they did in this field and why the movement to synergy dealt more with the synergistic interaction of language levels within the learner and not on the synergistic interaction of the learner with extrinsic or extraneous factors. The focus in this discipline, therefore, was on the intrinsic faculty of language proficiency and the learner's capacity for language learning.

This difference between ESL's focus on extrinsic variables in language learning and SLP's focus on intrinsic variables did produce divergent theoretical and pedagogical implications.

This difference in emphasis between the two fields is easily noted when we compare some of the most recent theoretical discussions within these disciplines. In ESL, for example, Bernard Spolsky (1988), has recently advanced an initial attempt to detail a general theory of second language learning. While there are numerous interesting aspects of his proposal, two issues stand out in light of the previous discussion. First, he has attempted to build into his model a range of variability. He suggests a need to recognize that there are no pedagogical panaceas, that there are many ways that learners may develop a second language, and that this flexibility is primarily due to a complex collection of typical and categorical rules or conditions that must be considered. Language learning, he suggests, results from the interaction and integration of a large number of factors and not from any single factor.

Besides this emphasis on theoretical and pedagogical flexibility, the second issue of interest involves the variables (or factors) he attempts to account for in his theory. The theoretical framework consists of several factoral clusters which must be considered:

(1) Knowledge and skills at the moment (including L1 and L2 knowledge),
(2) Intrinsic faculties (including physiological, biological, intellectual, and cognitive skills),
(3) Affective factors (personality, attitudes, motivations, and anxiety), and

(4) Opportunity (including exposure, pedagogical technique, and some sociological factors).

In fact, Spolsky claims that there are 75 (or fewer or more) preference conditions that need to be considered. Here we see an emphasis on factors or variables other than just the learner's intrinsic language learning capacity.

In contrast to Spolsky's theory that attempts to build in variation and incorporate a number of variables into a theory of language learning, the most recent theoretical discussion in speech-language pathology focuses exclusively on the learner's intrinsic language abilities. This second theoretical discussion is advanced by David Crystal (1987) in the Journal of Clinical Linguistics and Phonetics. In this article, Crystal discusses "the current orthodoxy of breaking a patient's language down into levels ..." (1987:8). In this practice, language disability is defined according to problems within distinct language levels. Crystal suggests that a new theoretical approach considering the interactions between language levels be used to define language disability. Here is a support for synergy within the learner's system. To quote Crystal, mutal influence between some level exists, and

> this factor should play a more dominant role in our search for a general explanation of language handicap. (1987:20).

The point of interest for our purposes is that Crystal does not discuss or include the interaction or importance of extrinsic factors in his theory. Regardless of his actual beliefs, his expressed theory deals only with the intrinsic language system. This is a common phenomenon in speech-language pathology.

To summarize, both fields are similar in their objectives and their histories but they have had different areas of focus. Importantly, these differences have definite theoretical and pedagogical implications. In ESL, there has been a greater concern for theoretical foundations, a greater emphasis on variation, and a real attempt to consider extrinsic factors like affective variables, sociological variables, and access variables as an integral part of language learning, assessment, and teaching.

In speech-language pathology, the emphasis on the intrinsic faculty necessary for learning and the focus on the individual learner has resulted in the development of effective techniques for individual language intervention, the utilization of methodological innovations like single subject research paradigms, and a greater emphasis on the role of neuroscience in language learning and teaching.

The Fourth Modification: Professional Synergy

Given the similar evolution of these two disciplines and the different focuses that they maintained, it is clear that each discipline possesses different strengths and advantages regarding the re-establishment of their emphasis on synergy. These mutual interests and complementary differences should result in a fourth modification within the evolution of these fields of applied linguistics. They should create a professional synergy in order to mutually benefit from one another. Speech-language pathology can utilize the work in ESL to become less intrinsically or faculty oriented and can start focusing on extrinsic variables. This is necessary given the fact that current research demonstrates that many children are mis-identified as having intrinsic language disorders when they are merely normal language learners with cultural or linguistic differences. The ESL focus on sociological and access variables will aid the speech-language pathologist in becoming more effective in the valid identification of language disorders in diverse populations. In general, speech-language pathologists are naive regarding applied linguistic principles and theoretical foundations. The interaction with ESL will also enable the field of speech-language pathology to become more theory driven and more linguistically sophisticated.

The discipline of ESL can also benefit from this interaction. By utilizing the individualized pedagogical techniques developed in speech-language pathology, ESL teachers may increase their effectiveness. When dealing with accent fossilization, for example, some of the individualized intervention techniques developed in speech-language pathology may be particularly effective. ESL can also benefit from the emphasis that speech-language pathology has placed on single subject research paradigms. Based on concerns regarding treatment efficacy, researchers in speech-language pathology have developed numerous single subject designs can be effectively applied in ESL research. Finally, as theoretical models involving Parallel Distributive Processing (Rummelhart and McClelland 1986) and other neuroscientific data are presented in applied linguistics as support for theories and pedagogical innovations, ESL can benefit from speech-language pathology's greater sophistication in neuroscientific research and theory. This will enable ESL professionals to become better consumers of these theoretical and pedagogical innovations.

In 1982 Buckminster Fuller commented on the movement toward hyperspecialization in our culture (Fuller 1982). Just as with extreme biological specialization, he stated that professional hyperspecialization has significant negative consequences including isolation, futility, confusion, and loss of effectiveness. As recommended by Fuller, the disciplines involved with applied linguistic issues must interact with one another to share knowledge, experience, and insight. Synergy is not just a concept applied appropriately to linguistics. It should also be applied to linguists.

References

Abkarian, G.G. 1977. "The Changing Face of a Discipline: Isn't it 'Romantic'?" *Journal of Speech and Hearing Disorders* 42.422-435.

Albrechtsen, et al. 1979.

Bachman, L. and A. Palmer. 1983. "The Construct Validity of FSI Oral Interview". *Issues in Language Testing Research* ed. by J.W. Oller, Jr., 154-169. Rowley, MA: Newbury House.

Bloomfield, L. 1933. *Language*. New York: Holt, Rinehart and Winston.

Bloomfield, L. 1939. *Linguistic Aspects of Science. International Encyclopedia of Unified Science, Vol 1, No. 4.* Chicago: University of Chicago Press.

Blue, C.M. 1975. "The Marginal Communicator". *Language, Speech, and Hearing Services in Schools* 6.32-37.

Brown, G. and G. Yule. 1983. *Teaching the Spoken Language*. Cambridge: Cambridge University Press.

Bruton, A. and V. Samuda. 1980. "Learner and Teacher Roles in the Treatment of Oral Error in Group Work". *RELC Journal.*

Carroll, J.B. 1961. "Fundamental Considerations in Testing for English Language Proficiency of Foreign Students". *Testing*, 31-40. Washington, DC: Center for Applied Linguistics.

Carroll. J.B. 1983. "Psychometric Theory and Language Testing". *Issues in language testing research* ed. by J.W. Oller, 80-107. Rowley, MA: Newbury House.

Corder, P. 1973. *Introducing Applied Linguistics*. Harmondsworth: Penguin.

Crystal, D. 1987. "Towards a 'Bucket' Theory of Language Disability: Taking Account of Interaction between Linguistic Levels". *Clinical Linguistics and Phonetics* 1.7-22.

Drake, G. 1977. "American Linguistic Prescriptionism: Its Decline and Revival in the 19th Century". *Language in Society* 6.323-340.

Fanselow, J.F. 1977. "The Treatment of Error in Oral Work". *Foreign language Annals* 10.583-593.

Ferguson, C. 1977. "Simplified Registers, Broken Language and Gastarbeiter Deutsch". *Deutsch im Kontakt mit anderen Sprachen* ed. by C. Molony, H. Zobl and W. Stolting, 25-39. Kronberg Ts: Scriptor.

Ferguson, C. and C. E. de Bose. 1977. "Simplified Registers, Broken Language and Pidginization. *Pidgin and creole linguistics* ed. by A. Valdman, 99-125. Bloomington: Indiana University Press.

Fries, C.C. 1952. *The Structure of English*. New York: Harcourt, Brace, and Company.

Fuller, R.B. 1982. *Synergetics*. New York: McMillian.

Gardner, R.C. 1985. *Social Psychology and Second Language Learning: The Role of Attitudes and Motivation*. London: Edward Arnold.

Gardner, R.C. and W.E. Lambert. 1972. *Attitudes and Motivation in Second Language Learning*. Rowley, MA; Newbury House.

Guiora, A.Z. et al. 1972. The Effects of Benziodiazepine (Valium) on Permeability of Language Ego Boundaries. *Language Learning* 30.351-363.

Johansson, S. 1975. *Papers in Contrastive Linguistics and Language Testing*. Lund: C.K.W. Gleerup

Klein, W. 1986. *Second Language Acquisition*. Cambridge: Cambridge University Press.

Krashen, S. 1981. *Second Language Acquisition and Second Language Learning*. Oxford: Pergamon Press.

Lado, R. 1961. *Language Testing*. New York: McGraw Hill.

Lee, L. and G. Canter. 1971. "Developmental Sentence Scoring: A Clinical Procedure for Estimating Syntactic Development in Children 's Spontaneous Speech". *Journal of Speech and Hearing disorders* 36.315-340.

Leonard, L.B. 1972. "What is Deviant Language?" *Journal of Speech and Hearing Disorders* 37.427-446.

Lerea, L. 1958. "Assessing Language Development". *Journal of Speech and Hearing Research* 1.75-85.

Lieberman, L.R. 1965. "The Boy Who Wouldn't Say "huh": A Suggested Area for Research". *Journal of Speech and Hearing Disorders* 30.184-186.

Monsees, E.K. and C. Berman. 1968. "Speech and Language Screening in a Summer Headstart Program". *Journal of Speech and Hearing Disorders* 33.121-126.

Muma. 1975.

Newmeyer, F. 1980. *Linguistic Theory in America*. New York: Academic Press.

Oller, J.W., Jr. 1973. "Pragmatic Language Testing". *Language Sciences* 28.7-12.

Oller, J.W., Jr. 1979. *Language Tests at School*. London: Longman.

Oller, J.W., Jr. and P. Richard-Amato. 1983. *Methods That Work*. Rowley, MA: Newbury House.

Palmer, A.S. 1978. "Measurements of Achievement, Communication, Incorporation and Integration for Two Classes of Formal ESL Learners". Paper read at the Fifth International Congress of Applied Linguistics, Montreal, Canada.

Panagos, J.M. 1974. "String Complexity Increases Phonemic Interference". *Perceptual and Motor Skills* 38. 1219-1222.

Prutting, C.A. 1979. "Process /pras/ses/n: the Action of Moving Forward from One Point to Another on the Way to Completion". *Journal of Speech and Disorders* 44.3-30.

Rees, N. 1979. "Breaking Out of the Centrifuge". *American Speech-Language-Hearing Association* 21.992-997.

Rees, N. and Shulmann. 1978. "I Don't Understand What You Mean by Comprehension". *Journal of Speech and Hearing Disorders* 43.208-219.

Robbins, S.D. 1933. "Relation between the Short Auditory Memory Span Disability and Disorders of Speech". *Proceedings of the American Society for Study of Disorders of Speech* 3.9-15.

Rosenberg, P.E. 1966. "Misdiagnosis of Children with Auditory Problems". *Journal of Speech and Hearing Disorders* 31.279-283.

Rumelhart, D.E., J.L. McClelland and the PDP Research Group 1986. *Parallel Distributive Processing: Explorations in the Microstructures of Cognition: Vol. 1. Foundations*. Cambridge: MIT Press. Scargill, M.H. 1954. "Modern Linguistics and Recovery from Aphasia". *Journal of Speech and Hearing Disorders* 19. 507-513.

Schumann, J.H. 1978. "The Acculturation Model for Second-language Acquisition". *Second Language Acquisition and Foreign Language Teaching* ed. by R. Gingras, 27-50. Arlington, VA: Center for Applied Linguistics.

Shriner, T.H., M.S. Holloway and R.G. Daniloff. 1969. "The Relationship between Articulatory Deficits and Syntax in Speech Defective Children". *Journal of Speech and Hearing Research* 12.319-325

Siegel, G. 1967. "Interpersonal Approaches to the Study of Communication Disorders". *Journal of Speech and Hearing Disorders* 32.221-230.

Spolsky, B. 1968. "Language Testing — The Problem of Validation". *TESOL Quarterly* 2.88-94.

Spolsky, B. 1978. "Linguists and Language Testers". *Advances in Language Testing: Series 2, Approaches to Language Testing* ed. by B. Spolsky. Arlington, VA: Center for Applied Linguistics.

Spolsky, B. 1988. "Bridging the Gap: A General Theory of Second Language Learning". *TESOL Quarterly* 22.377-396.

Strauss, A.A. and A.A. McCarus. 1958. "A Linguist Looks at Aphasia in Children". *Journal of Speech and Hearing Disorders* 23.54-58.

Streng, A.H. 1972. *Syntax, Speech, and Hearing*. New York: Grune and Stratton.

Thomas. C.K. 1957. "Review of Henry L. Smith's 'Linguistic Science and the Teaching of English'." *Journal of Speech and Hearing Disorders* 22.398.

Travis, L.E. and B.J. Rasmus. 1931. "The Speech-sound Discrimination Ability of Cases with Functional Disorders of Articulation". *Quarterly Journal of Speech Education* 17.217- 226.

Tyack, D. 1972. "The Use of Language Samples in Clinical Settings". *PRCLD* 4.163-168.

Upshur, J.A. 1967. "English Language Tests and Prediction of Academic Success". *Selected Conference Papers of the Association of Teachers of English as a Second Language*. National Association for Foreign Student Affairs.

Upshur, J.A. and Homburg, T.J. 1983. "Some Relations among Language Tests at Successive Ability Levels". *Issues in Language Testing Research* ed. by J.W. Oller, Jr., 188-202. Rowley, MA: Newbury House.

Upshur, J.A. and A.S. Palmer. 1974. "Measurement of Accuracy, Communicativity, and Social Judgements for Two Classes of Foreign Language Speakers". *Selected papers from the Third International Congress of Applied Linguistics*, vol 2 ed. by A. Vredoodt. Heidelberg: Julius Gross.

Valette, R.M. 1964. "The Use of Dictee in the French Language Classroom". *TESOL Quarterly* 39.431-343.

Weiss, A.P. 1925. "Linguistics and Psychology". *Language* 1.52-57.

Weiner, P.S. 1967. "Auditory Discrimination and Articulation". *Journal of Speech and Hearing Disorders* 32.19-28.

Wilkins, D.A. 1976. *Notional Syllabus*. London: Oxford.

Woobert, C. 1920. "Pathological Conditions, Speech Defects". *Quarterly Journal of Speech Education* 6.62-75.

Phonological Aspects of Emerging Grammars

Judith A. Gierut
Indiana University

Phonological Aspects of Emerging Grammars

Speech-language pathology faces a serious dilemma as it enters the year 2000. On the one hand, one-third of clinical caseloads will involve teaching nonnative speakers of English (ASHA 1989). On the other, speech-language pathologists typically have little to no training in second language learning or instruction. An obvious and immediate solution to the problem is to merely apply tried-and-true methods to this new population. However, in doing so, the assumption that grammars, learning patterns, and methods of instruction are comparable across language learning populations must be accepted. On prima facie grounds, this assumption does not seem unreasonable. Speech disordered clients and second language learners are both involved in the process of acquiring the ambient language. For both groups, the clinician must initially determine what the speaker already knows about the target grammar and what still remains to be learned, and then must develop and implement effective ways of teaching these novel aspects of grammar. On empirical grounds, however, this assumption remains wholly untested. The relationship between speech disorders and second language learning has not been established and only very recently has it even been considered a potential area of investigation (Gierut 1988).

Clearly, speech-language pathology has much to learn from the study of second language acquisition and instruction; even so, this contribution is not unidirectional. There are mutual benefits to be gained from a sharing of theoretical and applied information between these two disciplines. One unique way in which speech-language pathology can contribute to the area of second language acquisition is through its application and understanding of a well-founded, flexible experimental paradigm: the single-subject design (McReynolds and Kearns 1983). This paradigm has been used extensively in applied and behavioral sciences including, for example, clinical psychology, education and special education, audiology and speech-language pathology. The single-subject paradigm is not to be confused with the case study, an approach that fails to recognize basic principles of research such as the definition and systematic manipulation of variables (Hersen and Barlow 1976). This paradigm also overcomes limitations of large group designs such as heterogeneity of a population. Furthermore, it directly addresses issues second language researchers have been concerned with, such as the identification of individual learning strategies in the face of discovering more general patterns of learning consistent across subjects and the classroom application of research results (Lightbown 1985). Despite advantages of single-subject designs, second language researchers have rarely employed this paradigm. In fact, even a most recent text on experimental paradigms for second language research has failed to cite even one single-subject design (Brown 1988).

Thus, the purpose of this paper is to explore the interconnections of speech disordered and second language learning populations by way of empirical investigations that use single-subject paradigms. This issue will be examined specific to the phonological systems of children learning to correct functional speech sound errors and adults learning the phonological system of a second language. These subgroups were selected for comparison because they present no organic or neurological involvement and exhibit emerging sound systems aimed at approximating the target system. Three specific cases will be examined: (1) the nature of the learner's grammar, (2) ease of learning during instruction, and (3) methods of teaching. At first glance, these subgroups of learners will appear to be different on all three counts; however, closer inspection will reveal that the limits of these potential differences must be more specifically delineated through controlled single-subject experimental research. Moreover, such research will have significant theoretical and pedagogical implications for both disciplines, speech-language pathology and second language instruction.

Nature of the Learner's Grammar

An obvious place to begin an empirical assessment of the similarities and differences among speech disordered children and second language learners is with the nature and structure of the phonological system. For the speech disordered child, current research has supported phonological descriptions that are independent of the target or adult phonology as developed within a standard generative framework (Camarata and Gandour 1984; Dinnsen 1984; Dinnsen, Chin, Elbert, and Powell 1990; Dinnsen and Maxwell 1981; Gierut 1986b, 1989a; Maxwell 1981; Williams and Dinnsen 1987). These descriptions are in contrast to those that establish 1:1 correspondences between child and adult systems as developed within natural process (Hodson 1980; Ingram 1976, 1981; Shriberg and Kwiatkowski 1980; Weiner 1979) or place-voice-manner frameworks (Turton 1973; Weber 1970).

Thus far, the sound systems of more than 90 preschool children with phonological disorders have been examined in two major ongoing research projects at Indiana University (Elbert and Dinnsen, "Phonological knowledge and learning patterns"; Gierut, "Learnability of sound systems"). For each child, qualitative descriptions of the phonetic and phonemic inventories, distribution of sounds, use of phonological rules, positional and inventory constraints, and underlying representations of morphemes were developed (cf. Chomsky and Halle 1968; Dinnsen 1984; Gierut 1986a; Kenstowicz and Kisseberth 1979). The qualitative descriptions were based upon extended samples of spontaneous connected speech and single-word elicited productions following procedures outlined by Gierut (1985). Then, for purposes of experimental treatment, it was necessary to determine how these independent phonological descriptions related to the ambient phonology. In other words, how did each child's grammar compare to the target grammar? What did a child know about the target grammar? Toward this end, a quantitative metric for translating the qualitative phonological descriptions was developed (Dinnsen 1986). The quantitative metric was a weighted calculation, independent of the nature or size of the speech sample obtained, whereby points were assigned for production and appropriate use of sounds in specific contexts as associated with the generative descriptions. Points were tallied and percentages calculated to determine what proportion of the entire phonology was attributable to particular phonological properties and phenomena. From the qualitative and quantitative analyses combined, the nature and boundaries of disordered phonological systems were then described.

A first observation that emerged from these analyses was that speech disordered children's phonologies could be described by five independent qualitative categories: (1) sounds that were ambient-like or essentially correct in all respects; (2) sounds that were produced in error as a result of the misapplication of phonological rules (i.e., either the use of rules that were not target-appropriate, such as postvocalic glottalization or deletion, or the nonuse of rules that were target-appropriate, such as intervocalic flapping); (3) sounds that occurred in some positions but not others as accounted for by a positional constraint; (4) emerging sounds that were very low in frequency of occurrence and often in free variation with other sounds; and (5) sounds that were excluded from both the phonetic and phonemic inventories (Dinnsen, Elbert, and Weismer 1980; Gierut 1985; Gierut, Elbert, and Dinnsen 1987).

A second observation was that the average disordered phonological system structured much like the display shown in Figure 1. Figure 1 is a composite phonology based on the qualitative and quantitative analyses of 40 speech disordered subjects (Dinnsen 1986). Approximately one third of an average speech disordered phonology was associated with essentially target-appropriate sound productions in all contexts. Errors that did occur derived, for the most part, from constraints on the inventory (30%) followed by phonological rules (20%). Collapsing even further, an average speech disordered phonology was characterized by approximately 60% ambient-like underlying representations (i.e., ambient and phonological rules combined) and 40% nonambient-like underlying representations (i.e., positional plus emerging plus inventory). This characterization suggests that, contrary to frequent claims (for review, see Ingram 1976; Leonard 1985; Stoel-Gammon and Dunn 1985), children with phonological disorders have errors originating primarily from incorrect underlying representations rather than from phonological rules. Consequently, the major problem facing the child in treatment appears to be one of restructuring lexical representations.

In a recent pilot study, similar qualitative and quantitative analyses were conducted for second language learners as a means of characterizing an average interlanguage phonology (Gierut, Dinnsen, and Bardovi-Harlig 1987). Exactly the same procedures described for speech disordered children were followed, however, a much smaller population of language learning subjects was sampled. In this pilot study, three subjects were examined: two were of the same native language background (i.e., Chinese, Wu dialect) and one spoke another native language (i.e., Arabic, Gulf dialect). The average interlanguage characterization, shown in Figure 2, was generally consistent with each individual subject's emerging phonology. As with

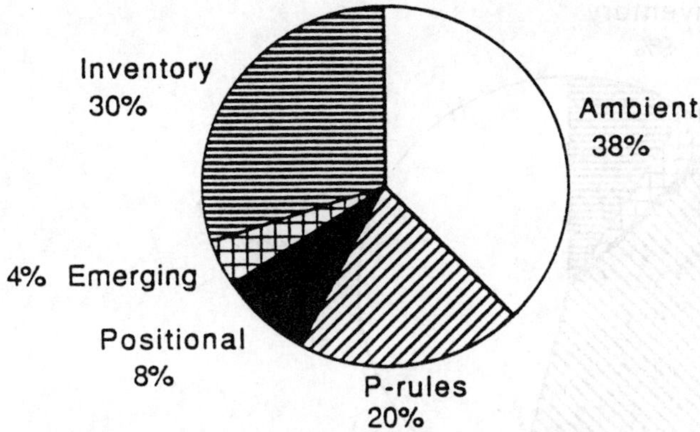

Figure 1. Composite speech disordered phonology based on qualitative and quantitative analyses of 40 speech disordered children (from Dinnsen 1986).

disordered phonologies, the largest portion of an interlanguage was associated with target-like productions (46%) and the majority of errors were associated with inventory constraints and phonological rules. However, in contrast, phonological rules were twice as prevalent for second language learners as for speech disordered children (41% versus 20%); whereas, inventory constraints accounted for less than 10% of the interlanguage phonology versus 30% for speech disordered children. For the second language learner, then, errors appear to result primarily from the application of phonological rules on correct underlying representations. This implies that, in contrast to speech disordered children, changing phonological rules will be a more significant problem for the second language learner. Although consistent with current second language learning literature (Dickerson, L. J. 1975; Dickerson, W. B. 1976, 1987; Eckman 1981; Flege 1987; Hammerly 1982), these observations are limited and may be an artifact of examining the interlanguages of speakers whose native languages are comprised of relatively large consonantal inventories thereby precluding a higher incidence of inventory constraints.

This initial comparison suggests that, while the grammars of phonologically disordered children and second language learners can be described by the same phonological categories, the organization of these grammars may not be identical or even equivalent. In training, then, the learner's task of altering the existing grammar to be more in line with the target may also be very different.

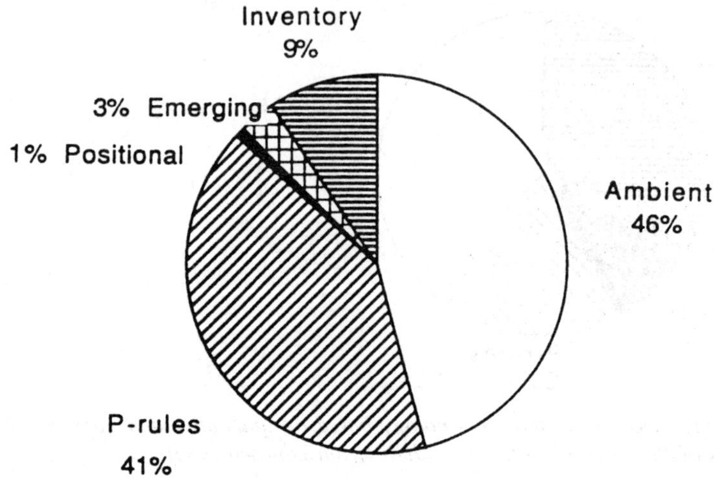

Figure 2. Composite interlanguage phonology based on qualitative and quantitative analyses of 3 adults learning English as a second language (from Gierut, Dinnsen, and Bardovi-Harlig 1987).

Ease of Learning During Instruction

This leads to the second point of examination: that of establishing ease of phonological learning during instruction. Will the differences observed in phonological organization across populations play a role in learning? Are the phonological differences psychologically real? In other words, will these differences have behavioral consequences during instruction and, further, will these differences be reflected in differential patterns of learning for the two populations?

For the speech disordered child, learning during treatment has been directly linked to the child's existing knowledge of the target sound system (Dinnsen and Elbert 1984; Elbert, Dinnsen, and Powell, 1984; Gierut and Dinnsen 1987; Gierut et al. 1987). For this population, the nature of a child's underlying representation — either correct or incorrect — has been shown to influence ease of learning. Specifically, in a single-subject multiple probe, multiple baseline study, six phonologically disordered children received instruction on various errored aspects of their sound systems (Gierut et al. 1987). Children were assigned to one of two experimental groups. One group of three children first received treatment on aspects of the target grammar of which they had least knowledge. In general, these were sounds excluded from a child's phonetic and phonemic inventories, that is, those sounds with nonambient-like underlying representations. The other group of three children first received treatment on aspects of the target grammar of which they had most knowledge, or sounds in error as a result of the application of phonological rules (i.e., ambient-like underlying representations). All children received treatment on three errored aspects of their sound system, ranging from most to least knowledge or vice versa. Throughout treatment, changes in the accuracy of production of these sounds were monitored.

Results indicated that, regardless of the starting point of treatment (most versus least knowledge), all children demonstrated a similar pattern of learning. As represented in Figures 3 and 4, a child's performance on sounds in error as a result of phonological rules (open circles) was always as good or better than performance on sounds in error as a result of constraints on the inventory (closed squares). To put it another way, learning to alter phonological rules was easier for speech disordered children than learning new sounds that were not previously in the inventory. Apparently, restructuring the lexicon was a difficult task for these children.

A second unexpected but interesting finding emerged regarding starting point of treatment. For children who began treatment with sounds affected by phonological rules (Figure 3), change in the phonological system was limited and well-defined. Little to no improvements were evidenced in sounds of which these children had least knowledge (closed squares). Quite a different pattern of learning emerged for children who first received treatment on sounds excluded from the inventory (Figure 4). In this condition, global improvements on all previously errored aspects of the system were evidenced. How was it that the payoffs for these children were greater even though they were presented with the more difficult problem of restructuring their lexicon? A comparable demonstration involving the acquisition of mathematical skills may help to interpret these unusual findings (Yao 1989). Consider a child who does not know how to perform the operations of addition, subtraction, multiplication, or division. If this child is first taught division, he or she will not only learn to divide but also, by implication and necessity to this operation, to add, subtract, and multiply. On the other hand, if this child is first taught addition, he or she will learn this specific operation, but nothing about learning addition will neces-

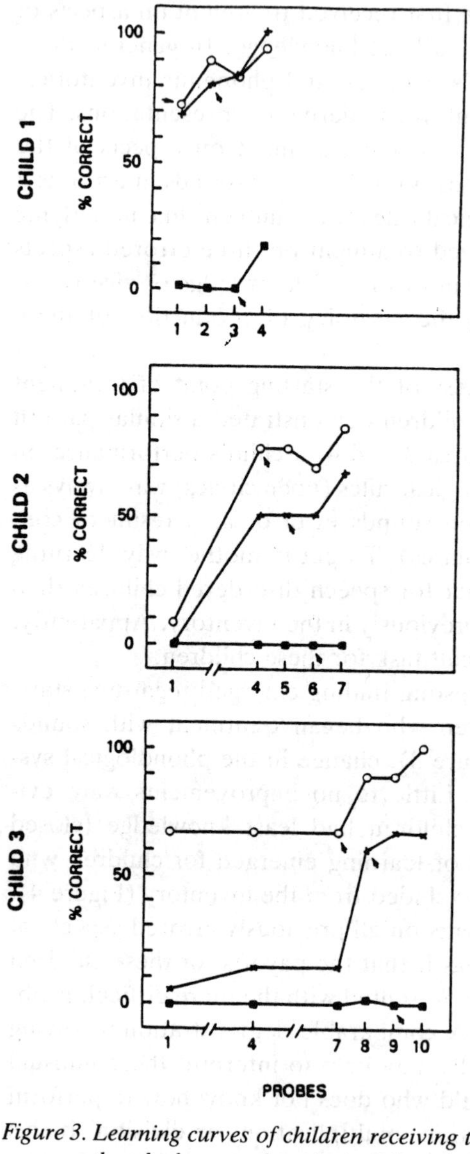

Figure 3. Learning curves of children receiving treatment beginning with sounds of which they had most phonological knowledge (from Gierut, Elbert, and Dinnsen, 1987). Open circles signify properties of the phonology of which a child had most knowledge; closed squares signify properties of which a child had least knowledge.

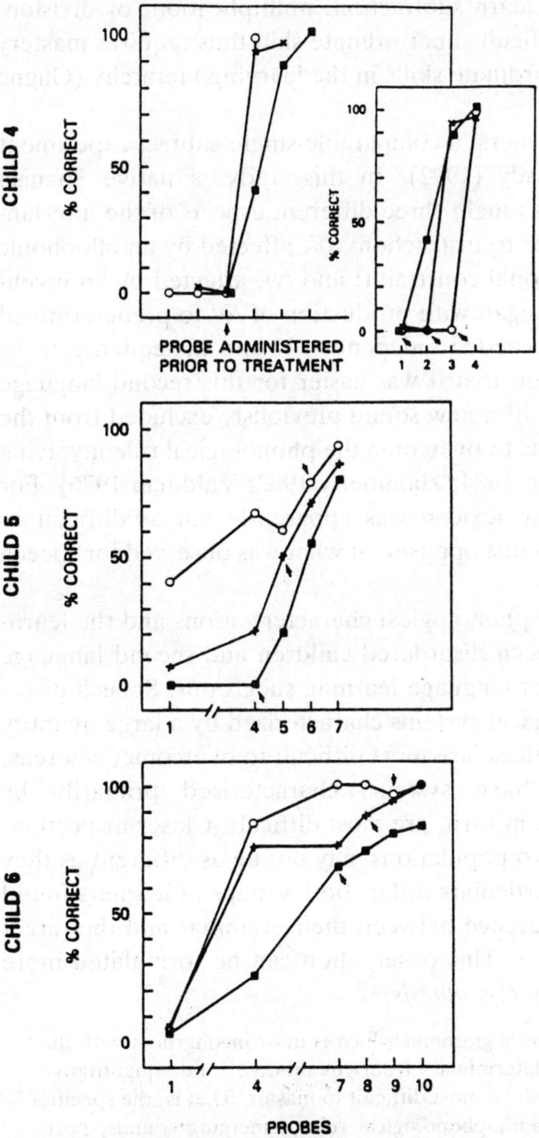

Figure 4. Learning curves of children receiving treatment beginning with sounds of which they had least phonological knowledge (from Gierut, Elbert, and Dinnsen 1987). As in Figure 3, open circles indicate most knowledge; closed squares indicate least knowledge.

sarily lead the child to also learn subtraction, multiplication, or division. Performance of the more difficult superordinate skill thus requires mastery of other coordinate and subordinate skills in the learning hierarchy (Gagne 1968, 1977).

For second language learners, a comparable single-subject experiment has been conducted by Hardy (1992). In this study, a native Spanish speaker learning English was taught three different aspects of the interlanguage that were in error prior to instruction: /ð/, affected by an allophonic rule; /z/, affected by a positional constraint; and /v/, affected by an inventory constraint. Instruction began with production of /ð/ to predetermined criterion levels and then proceeded independently and in sequence to /z/ and then /v/. Results indicated that it was easier for this second language learner to master production of a new sound previously excluded from the inventory (i.e., /v/) than it was to overcome the phonological rule involving /ð/ (cf. Flege and Hillenbrand 1984; Hammerly 1982; Valdman 1976). For this learner, restructuring the lexicon was apparently not as difficult as altering phonological rules — just opposite of what was observed for speech disordered children.

At first glance, both the phonological characterizations and the learning patterns suggest that speech disordered children and second language learners may be very different language learning subgroups. Speech disordered children have phonological systems characterized by a large quantity of inventory constraints and these are most difficult to overcome; whereas, second language learners have systems characterized primarily by phonological rules and these, in turn, are most difficult. Closer inspection, however, suggests that the two populations may not be as different as they first appear. Although the particulars differ, both groups of learners found that the area of greatest difference between their grammar and the target grammar was hardest to learn. This observation can be formulated more specifically as the *Congruency Hypothesis*:

> That property of a learner's grammar which is most incongruent with the target grammar, as determined from qualitative and quantitative phonological analyses, will be most difficult to master. That is, the specific phonological property (i.e., phonological rules, emerging sounds, positional or inventory constraints) that accounts for the greatest proportion of errors in a learner's grammar will be hardest to overcome. It is the *magnitude* of this difference between qualitative properties of the learner's grammar versus the target grammar that will influence ease of learning.

Many implications and experimental questions derive from this hypothesis. The Congruency Hypothesis suggests that the linguistic account of errors is merely a descriptive statement that has little impact on learning; rather, learning is governed by the magnitude of this account. In other words, the specific nature of the language problem may not be as important as establishing the extent of that problem. Phonological rules, for example, may not be the linguistic factor that makes learning difficult for the second language learner. It may simply be that a greater proportion of rules operate in the learner's interlanguage relative to other phonological properties. Similarly, for the speech disordered child, inventory constraints may be especially difficult but only because the greatest magnitude of difference between the child's grammar and the target is attributable to this aspect of the phonology.

This implication has a further consequence of removing language learning (or at least this aspect of learning) from a linguistic domain and placing it in a cognitive domain, on par with mastery of other complex processes and skills. From this perspective, why should a lack of congruency with the target grammar be a recognizable problem for the language learner? How is it possible that the language learner is able to detect areas and varying magnitudes of difference among grammars? Perhaps, the learner is able to access cognitively a congruency metric whereby scaler dimensions can be identified. This type of cognitive ability is not unusual and has been demonstrated in other complex processing domains such as vision (e.g., big/little), audition (e.g. loud/soft), tactile (e.g., rough/smooth), or gustation (e.g., sour/sweet) (Smith 1984; Smith and Kemler 1977). In principle, then, it is at least plausible that a learner can detect magnitudes of difference along linguistic dimensions as well.

One important feature of the Congruency Hypothesis is that individual differences are tolerated. Both within and across populations, any given speaker may find different aspects of their phonology more or less congruent with the target and, therefore, easier or more difficult to learn. Furthermore, any two speakers displaying exactly the same type of error relative to the target grammar may learn in different ways. To illustrate, consider two second language learners of the same native language background who also are acquiring the same target language. These two learners may display identical errors in production that derive from an allophonic rule. The formulation of this rule and its conditions for application are identical for both learners. With instruction, one learner may find this rule relatively easy to overcome. In line with the Congruency Hypothesis, this learner's interlanguage would likely be characterized by a relatively small proportion of phonological rules (regardless of the specific type of rule); other qualitative phonological properties (e.g., inventory constraints) would account for the majority of this learner's errors. In contrast, the other learner may experience great difficulty learning to overcome the same rule. Predictably, this learner's interlanguage would consist of a relatively large proportion of phonological rules, with few errors deriving from inventory or positional constraints. Thus, even though both learners may have had an identical pattern of error, they would be confronted with very different language learning problems given the magnitude of the error relative to other phonological properties operating in their system.

The Congruency Hypothesis also takes into account the fact that a learner's phonological system is in transition, that change and variation are to be expected. Thus, the magnitude of difference among grammars (or that phonological property which will be easier or more difficult to learn) will be continually modified as a learner's phonology emerges over time or with instruction.

Finally, the Congruency Hypothesis is unique from other linguistic proposals that attempt to account for ease of learning. For instance, the Congruency Hypothesis is different from the Contrastive Analysis Hypothesis for second language learners (Lado 1957). The Congruency Hypothesis does not derive from fixed 1:1 native-target language correspondences as does the Contrastive Analysis Hypothesis; rather, it is based on the interlanguage of an individual speaker. For instance, the Contrastive Analysis Hypothesis predicts that allophonic problems will be difficult uniformally for all second language learners of the same native language mastering the same target language. The Congruency Hypothesis, on the other hand, predicts that allophonic problems will be difficult for a given second language learner if and only if the magnitude of this problem exceeds other phonological difficulties that learner may encounter. In this case, one particular second language learner may find allophonic problems difficult, whereas another learner may not. The Congruency Hypothesis thus predicts variation in ease of learning for speakers of the same language background.

Although the Congruency Hypothesis provides a novel account of ease of language learning applicable to a variety of populations, its validity remains untested. One experimental means of evaluating this hypothesis involves the use of a multiple baseline across subjects design. Briefly, in this design, a first subject is enrolled in training, while performance of remaining subjects is monitored. When Subject 1 completes the training phase, training is then instated for Subject 2 and all other subjects are monitored. The multiple baseline thus consists of a sequence of observation and training. To demonstrate experimental control, changes in performance are expected only under conditions of training and not observation. Replications across subjects demonstrate the powerful effects of training variables and provide external validity to the findings.

As a first test of the Congruency Hypothesis, the following multiple baseline across subjects study is proposed. Two independent groups of subjects would be needed, with each group consisting of 6 learners (i.e., 12 learners in total): 3 speech disordered children and 3 second language learning adults. For each subject, only one errored aspect of their phonology would be trained, as identified uniquely from qualitative and quantitative phonological analyses of each learner's grammar. All subjects in one group would receive training on properties of their grammar that were errored but relatively congruent (in magnitude) with the target ("Congruent" group). For instance, this may be phonological rules for speech disordered children but inventory constraints for second language learners. All subjects in the second group would be trained on properties of their grammar that were errored but highly divergent (in magnitude) from the target — perhaps, inventory constraints for speech disordered children versus phonological rules for second language learners ("Incongruent" group). Both congruent and incongruent aspects of each learner's phonology would be monitored to determine how each subject changed his or her existing grammar with training.

A number of outcomes are possible. First, if the Congruency Hypothesis is correct, each experimental group ("Congruent" versus "Incongruent") would perform in different ways. However, members of a given experimental group would perform identically, be they speech disordered children or second language learning adults. Even though subjects would have likely received treatment on different phonological properties (e.g., phonological rules versus inventory constraints), those in the "Congruent" group would find learning easy in contrast to the "Incongruent" group where learning would be more difficult. Continuing along this line, if a given speech disordered child exhibited a phonological system with patterns characteristic of interlanguages (i.e., larger proportions of phonological rules), then this child's learning likewise would mirror that of the second language learning adult. This particular child would probably find that altering phonological rules is a difficult task. Vice versa, a second language learner with a greater proportion of inventory constraints presumably would find this aspect of phonology difficult to learn, much like a typical speech disordered child.

A second possible outcome would be that populations, not experimental groups, would perform similarly, supporting the conclusion that language learning is comparable within but not across populations. If this were the case, all speech disordered children would be expected to learn in comparable ways, regardless of the phonological property being trained or the relative magnitude of difference of this property from the target grammar. The same would be true for all second language learners; however, these learners as a group would perform differently than speech disordered children.

A third possibility is associated with the phonological property being taught. For all learners, overcoming phonological rules may be easier than inventory constraints. A finding of this type would imply that there are learning patterns characteristic of specific language structures and these would be distinct from patterns observed in other higher-order learning tasks. This finding would support the conclusion that language learning is not merely an instantiation of cognition, but is unique in its own right.

Finally, each learner could perform in a different way suggesting that individual learning styles supersede any general language learning strategies and, further, that there is no relationship among learners within the same population or across different populations. The implication here is that there are no common or predictable properties of language learning in particular and, possibly, the same would hold for learning in general.

It is easy to see that a study of this type has a potential impact for both disciplines, speech-language pathology and second language acquisition. The results of such a study may offer preliminary solutions to important problems both disciplines have been wrestling with for many decades. At the very least, new and innovative lines of investigation would be opened.

Methods of Instruction

The third and final point of concern relates to methods of instruction. This topic will be discussed with regard to a very specific problem, that of inducing phonemic splits. The restructuring of allophones as distinct phonemes has long been cited as one of the most pervasive and difficult aspects of phonological learning facing the second language learner (Lado 1957). Only recently has this exact same problem been of concern for speech disordered children. There have been at least four reported cases of children who exhibit phonological patterns characteristic of allophonic relationships, namely, complementary distribution among sounds (Camarata and Gandour 1984; Gierut 1986b; Williams and Dinnsen 1987; Wolfe, Blocker, and Simmons 1988). Each of these required inducing a phonemic split through some form of clinical intervention; however, in only one case was the necessary intervention program actually described or implemented (Gierut 1986b).

The subject of this study was a four-year old boy who exhibited complementary distribution among the fricatives [f] and [s]: [f] always and only occurred word-initially and [s], always and only postvocalically. A multiple baseline design across word positions was used in training, such that the child first received minimal pair contrast treatment of the /f/-/s/ distinction in one word position (i.e., postvocalic) while it was also being monitored in a second position (i.e., word-initial). Upon reaching a performance-based criterion in the treated position, training then shifted to the monitored position. From this experimental sequence, it was possible to trace longitudinally changes in the structure and function of these fricatives in the child's phonology and, following from this, to identify distinct stages in the process of effecting a phonemic split.

As shown in Figure 5, prior to treatment, the child presented an allophonic problem as evidenced by 0% production of [f] postvocalically and [s] word-initially and near 100% production of [f] word-initially and [s] postvocalically. Following treatment in the first context of the multiple baseline sequence, the allophonic condition was no longer present. The child's phonology was modified to include an optional neutralization rule to account for morphophonemic alternations between [f] and [s] in treated postvocalic contexts. Then, following treatment in the second context of the multiple baseline, the child's phonology was further expanded to no longer include allophonic or neutralizing rules. In all word positions (but not for all morphemes), /f/ and /s/ were distinctive and maintained independent phonemic status.

Importantly, this study showed that: (1) it was possible to teach a child to restructure allophones as phonemes; (2) the method of minimal pair contrasts was an effective approach to the problem; and (3) the successful

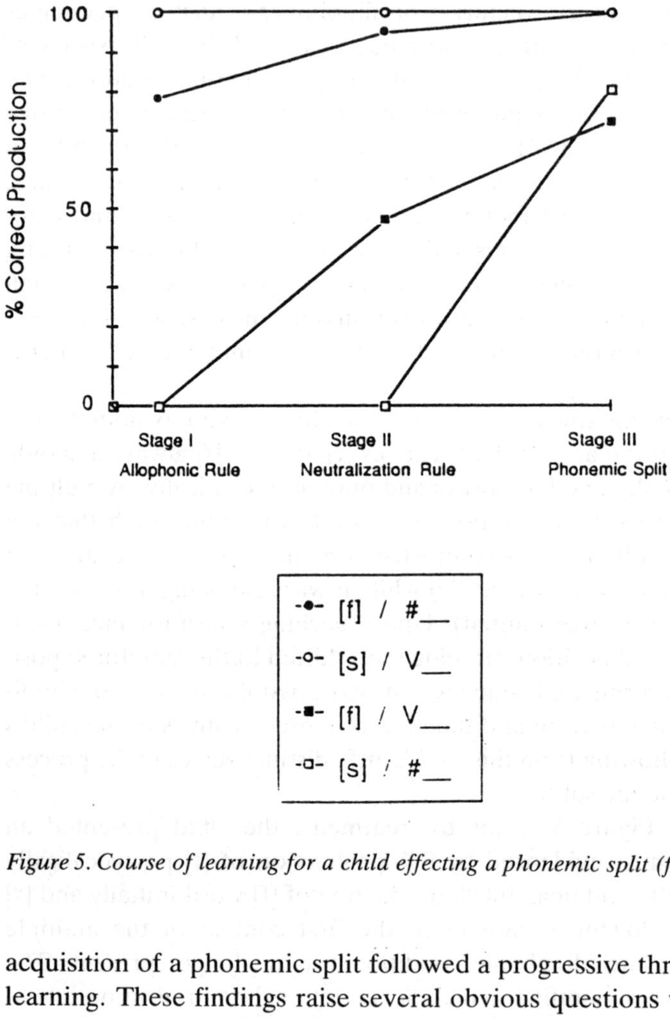

Figure 5. Course of learning for a child effecting a phonemic split (from Gierut 1986b).

acquisition of a phonemic split followed a progressive three-stage course of learning. These findings raise several obvious questions with regard to the second language learner. Can second language learners successfully restructure allophones as distinct phonemes as did this phonologically disordered child? Is the method of minimal pair contrasts an effective teaching approach to this end? Do second language learners follow similar stages in effecting phonemic splits? A systematic replication of this multiple baseline design with second language learning subjects will, in part, provide answers to these basic questions about the presumed difficulty second language learners have in restructuring allophones.

Yet, there is also a parallel line of research in speech-language pathology that may provide further insight into the nature of this problem. This line of research deals specifically with efficacy of treatment models. In particular, the results of a recent study on the efficacy of various models of phonological contrast treatment indicated that conventional minimal pair treatment had rather undesirable consequences on the phonological systems of some speech disordered children (Gierut 1990). Minimal pair treatment contributed to further collapses of phonemic distinctions in cases involving allophonic rules. In these instances, children seemed to focus on the similarities rather than the intended differences among the sounds being contrasted in treatment.

To illustrate, one particular child in this study substituted the palatal fricative [ʃ] in place of the target affricate /tʃ/ prior to treatment. This child also maintained an allophonic relationship between the palatal and velar fricatives, [ʃ] and [x], as evidenced by complementary distribution among these sounds: [ʃ] occurred prevocalically and [x] postvocalically. The child was subsequently enrolled in a remediation program involving minimal pair contrast treatment of the /tʃ/-/ʃ/ distinction. With treatment, the child learned to use the affricate [tʃ], but this sound was also produced in free variation with [ʃ] and [x]. In other words, all three of these sounds functioned as allophones of each other. Instead of adding /tʃ/ to his repertoire as a new contrastive phoneme, as was intended from the instruction, this child learned erroneously that [tʃ] was directly associated with [ʃ] as its variant. For some reason, the child equated, rather than differentiated, contrasts presented in the minimal pair approach.

Other models of phonological contrast treatment tested in this study did not show similar effects. For example, in the maximal opposition model (Gierut 1989b), contrasting sounds differed along multiple and broad dimensions of place, voice, and manner (e.g., /m/ versus /tʃ/). Here, a child's error substitutions were never a point of focus in sound pairs presented in treatment. Instead, the sound to be learned (e.g., /tʃ/) was only compared to a sound that the child already knew and was using appropriately and consistently in his or her existing phonology (e.g., /m/). Under conditions of this treatment, there were no instances of further collapses of phonemic distinctions for any children. This seemed to be the case because contrasting sounds were widely differentiated and were not intimately related to error substitutions but, rather, retained independent phonemic status in a child's grammar.

For second language learning, these findings offer a plausible hypothesis for a learner's difficulty in restructuring allophones as phonemes. Perhaps, the method of instruction constrains the second language learner's ability to effect a phonemic split. Minimal pair contrast training may not be the most appropriate teaching method for altering allophonic problems in this population, even though it is the logical and conventional choice (Lado, 1957). To test the accuracy of this hypothesis, a variety of phonological contrast treatment models, such as those currently available in speech-language pathology, must be tested as alternate or even preferred methods of instruction. The applicability of these models for changing aspects emerging phonological systems and for use with second language learners can be evaluated experimentally using another type of single-subject design, the alternating treatments design (Barlow and Hayes 1979). This design is well-suited to address this hypothesis because it allows for a comparison of the effects of two methods of instruction on a single subject. Both methods are presented and alternated in the same training phase. The subject discriminates between the two instructional methods and, consequently, performs differentially within each condition. The results of such research would make an important contribution to both speech-language pathology and second language instruction because the best methods of instruction for a given language learning population would be identified and, moreover, by comparison across populations, the conditions for applying each method would be determined.

Conclusion

This discussion and preliminary empirical study of the interrelationships between speech disordered children and second language learners has raised several important and timely research questions. The similarities gleaned from what appeared to be differences among these two populations underscore the necessity of cross-disciplinary interactions of an experimental nature. There is no doubt that the outcome of such interactions will have theoretical and applied significance for speech-language pathology, second language acquisition, and linguistics. From such interactions, the nature and boundaries of diverse language learning populations will be specified, the linguistic structures and processes characteristic of language learning will be characterized, and the necessary and specific properties of language will be delineated from those of cognition.

Acknowledgments

This research was supported in part by grants from the National Institutes of Health (DC 00433) and the Biomedical Research Support Grant Program (S07 RR 7031L) to Indiana University, Bloomington. I would like to thank Steve Chin, Phil Connell, Dan Dinnsen, Fred Eckman, and Jane Hardy for comments and suggestions on an earlier version of this manuscript.

References

American Speech-Language-Hearing Association. 1989. "Focus: Services in the schools". *ASHA* 31.37-70.

Barlow, D.H. and S.C. Hayes. 1979. "Alternating Treatments Design: One Strategy for Comparing the Effects of Two Treatments in a Single Subject". *Journal of Applied Behavior Analysis* 12.199-210.

Brown, J.D. 1988. *Understanding Research in Second Language Learning: A Teacher's Guide to Statistics and Research Design*. Cambridge: Cambridge University Press.

Camarata, S. and J. Gandour. 1984. "On Describing Idiosyncratic Phonologic Systems". *Journal of Speech and Hearing Disorders* 49.262-266.

Chomsky, N. and M. Halle. 1968. *The Sound Pattern of English*. New York: Harper and Row.

Dickerson, L.J. 1975. "The Learner's Interlanguage as a System of Variable Rules". *TESOL Quarterly* 9.401-407.

Dickerson, W.B. 1976. "The Psycholinguistic Unity of Language Learning and Language Change". *Language Learning* 26.215-231.

Dickerson, W.B. 1987. "Explicit Rules and the Developing Interlanguage Phonology". *Sound Patterns in Second Language Acquisition* ed. by A. James and J. Leather, 121-140. Dordrecht: Foris.

Dinnsen, D.A. 1984. "Methods and Empirical Issues in Analyzing Functional Misarticulations". Elbert, Dinnsen and Weismer 1984.5-17.

Dinnsen, D.A. 1986. "Fundamental Characteristics of Disordered Phonological Systems". Paper presented at the American Speech-Language-Hearing Association Convention, Detroit.

Dinnsen, D.A., S.B. Chin, M. Elbert, and T.W. Powell. 1990. "Some Constraints on Functionally Disordered Phonologies: Phonetic Inventories and Phonotactics". *Journal of Speech and Hearing Research* 33. 28-37.

Dinnsen, D.A. and M. Elbert. 1984. "On the Relationship between Phonology and Learning". Elbert, Dinnsen and Weismer 1984.59-68.

Dinnsen, D.A., M. Elbert and G. Weismer. 1980. "Some Typological Properties of Functional Misarticulation Systems". *Phonologica 1980* ed. by W.O. Dressler, 83-88. Innsbruck: Innsbrucker Beitrage Zur Sprachwissenschaft.

Dinnsen, D.A. and E.M. Maxwell. 1981. "Some Phonology Problems from Functional Speech Disorders". *Innovations in Linguistics Education* 2.79-98.

Eckman, F. 1981. "On the Naturalness of Interlanguage Phonological Rules". *Language Learning* 31.195-216.

Elbert, M., D.A. Dinnsen and T.W. Powell. 1984. "On the Prediction of Phonologic Generalization Learning Patterns". *Journal of Speech and Hearing Disorders* 49.309-317.

Elbert, M., D.A. Dinnsen and G. Weismer, eds. 1984. *Phonological Theory and the Misarticulating Child*. American Speech-Language-Hearing Association Monograph No. 22. Rockville, MD: American Speech-Language-Hearing Association.

Flege, J.E. 1987. "Effects of Equivalence Classification on the Production of Foreign Language Speech Sounds". James and Leather 1987.9-39.

Flege, J.E. and J. Hillenbrand. 1984. "Limits on Pronunciation Accuracy in Foreign Language Speech Production". *Journal of the Acoustical Society of America* 76.708-721.

Gagne, R.M. 1968. "Learning Hierarchies". *Educational Psychologist* 6.1-9.

Gagne, R.M. 1977. *The Conditions of Learning*. New York: Holt, Rinehart and Winston.

Gierut, J.A. 1985. *On the Relationship between Phonological Knowledge and Generalization Learning in Misarticulating Children*. Doctoral dissertation, Indiana University, Bloomington. Distributed by the Indiana University Linguistics Club, 1986.

Gierut, J.A. 1986a. "On the Assessment of Productive Phonological Knowledge". *NSSLHA Journal* 14. 83-101.

Gierut, J.A. 1986b. "Sound Change: A Phonemic Split in a Misarticulating Child". *Applied Psycholinguistics* 7.57-68.

Gierut, J.A. 1988. "Comparative Research on Language Learning". *Language Learning* 38.413-438.

Gierut, J.A. 1990. "Differential Learning of Phonological Oppositions". *Journal of Speech and Hearing Research* 33.540-549.

Gierut, J.A. 1989b. "Maximal Opposition Approach to Phonological Treatment". *Journal of Speech and Hearing Disorders* 54.9-19.

Gierut, J.A. 1989a. "Describing Developing Phonological Systems: A Surrebuttal". *Applied Psycholinguistics* 10.469-473.

Gierut, J.A. and D.A. Dinnsen. 1987. "On Predicting Ease of Phonological Learning". *Applied Linguistics* 8.35-57.

Gierut, J.A., D.A. Dinnsen and K. Bardovi-Harlig. 1987. "External Validity of Productive Phonological Knowledge: A First Report". *Research on Speech Perception Report* 13.241-248. Bloomington, IN: Speech Research Laboratory, Department of Psychology, Indiana University.

Gierut, J.A., M. Elbert and D.A. Dinnsen. 1987. "A Functional Analysis of Phonological Knowledge and Generalization Learning in Misarticulating Children". *Journal of Speech and Hearing Research* 30.462-479.

Hammerly, H. 1982. "Contrastive Phonology and Error Analysis". *International Review of Applied Linguistics* 20.17-32.

Hardy, J.E. 1992. "An Experimental Study of Phonological Learning in L2". This volume.

Hersen, M. and H.D. Barlow. 1976. *Single Case Experimental Designs: Strategies for Studying Behavior Change*. New York: Permagon Press.

Hodson, B.W. 1980. *The Assessment of Phonological Processes*. Danville, IL: Interstate Press.

Ingram, D. 1976. *Phonological Disability in Children*. New York: Elsevier.
Ingram, D. 1981. *Procedures for the Phonological Analysis of Children's Language*. Baltimore: University Park Press.
James, A. and J. Leather, eds. 1987. *Sound Patterns in Second Language Acquisition*. Dordrecht: Foris.
Kenstowicz, M. and C. Kisseberth. 1979. *Generative Phonology: Description and Theory*. New York: Academic Press.
Lado, R. 1957. *Linguistics Across Cultures*. Ann Arbor, MI: The University of Michigan Press.
Leonard, L.B. 1985. "Unusual and Subtle Phonological Behavior in the Speech of Phonologically Disordered Children". *Journal of Speech and Hearing Disorders* 50.4-13.
Lightbown, P. 1985. "Great Expectations: Second Language Acquisition Research and Classroom Teaching". *Applied Linguistics* 6.173-189.
Maxwell, E.M. 1981. *A Study of Misarticulation from a Linguistic Perspective*. Doctoral dissertation, Indiana University, Bloomington. Distributed by the Indiana University Linguistics Club, 1982.
McReynolds, L.V. and K.P. Kearns. 1983. *Single Subject Experimental Designs in Communicative Disorders*. Baltimore: University Park Press.
Shriberg, L.D. and J. Kwiatkowski. 1980. *Natural Process Analysis: A Procedure for the Phonological Analysis of Continuous Speech Samples*. New York: Wiley.
Smith, L. 1984. "Young Children's Understanding of Attributes and Dimensions: A Comparison of Conceptual and Linguistic Measures". *Child Development* 55.363-380.
Smith, L. and D. Kemler. 1977. "Developmental Trends in Free Classification: Evidence for a New Conceptualization of Perceptual Development". *Journal of Experimental Child Psychology* 24.279-298.
Stoel-Gammon, C. and C. Dunn. 1985. *Normal and Disordered Phonology in Children*. Austin, TX: PRO-ED.
Turton, C.J. 1973. "Diagnostic Implications of Articulation Testing". *Articulation and Learning* ed. by W.D. Wolfe and D.J. Goulding, 195-232. Springfield, IL: Charles C. Thomas.
Valdman, A. 1976. *Introduction to French Phonology and Morphology*. Rowley, MA: Newbury House.
Weber, J.L. 1970. "Patterning of Deviant Articulation Behavior". *Journal of Speech and Hearing Disorders* 35.135-141.
Weiner, F.F. 1979. *Phonological Process Analysis*. Baltimore: University Park Press.
Williams, A.L., and D.A. Dinnsen. 1987. "A Problem of Allophonic Variation in a Speech Disordered Child". *Innovations in Linguistic Education* 5.85-90.
Wolfe, V.I., S.D. Blocker and L. Simmons. 1988. "Consonant-vowel Interaction in an Idiosyncratic Phonologic System". Paper presented at the American Speech-Language-Hearing Association Convention, Boston.
Yao, K. 1989. *Acquisition of mathematical skills in a learning hierarchy by high and low ability students when instruction is omitted on coordinate and subordinate skills*. Unpublished doctoral dissertation, Indiana University, Bloomington.

Phonological Learning and Retention in Second Language Acquisition

Jane E. Hardy
Indiana University

Introduction

Predicting ease of phonological learning is a central research issue in both speech-language pathology and second language acquisition. It contributes to our understanding of how different populations learn sound systems, and is important for the structuring of effective and efficient teaching programs. Despite its theoretical and practical importance, there have been relatively few studies in either discipline that have directly addressed this issue. In speech-language pathology, Gierut and Dinnsen (1987) experimentally evaluated ease of learning for phonologically disordered children and demonstrated that errors involving sounds phonemically absent from the inventory were more difficult to overcome than errors resulting from phonological rules. In second language acquisition, Brière (1966) drew similar conclusions, while Hammerly (1982) found just the reverse, that errors resulting from phonological rules were more difficult to overcome than those resulting from inventory constraints (cf. Flege, 1987; Valdman, 1976). These conflicting findings from second language acquisition are limited since they derived from descriptive research that assumed homogeneity across the interlanguage (IL) phonological systems of L2 learners. The present study evaluates predictions regarding ease of phonological learning by employing controlled single-subject experimental methodologies common to speech-language pathology while focusing on the acquisition process by a second language learner.

Methods

Subject

The learner in this study was a 25-year old male native Spanish speaker from Madrid, Spain. He had a large vocabulary, advanced grammatical knowledge, and strong listening comprehension skills in English as demonstrated by a TOEFL score of 489, but he had comparatively poor English pronunciation. He had been enrolled in English courses prior to arrival in the United States, and was enrolled in intensive English language classes for six months while residing in the United States.

Phonological Analysis Prior to Training

A standard generative phonological analysis was developed prior to training, following procedures described by Kenstowicz and Kisseberth (1979). The analysis was based on two types of spontaneous speech: (1) connected speech elicited in conversation about the learner's future goals and plans for his stay in the United States; and (2) single words elicited in a picture-naming task involving a modification of a protocol developed by Gierut (1985) for use with phonologically disordered children. This protocol specifically sampled each target English sound in each relevant word position in a variety of exemplars, and also provided an opportunity for the learner to produce potential minimal pairs and morphophonemic alternations, critical forms of evidence for establishing phonemic contrasts and phonological rules. Speech samples were audio recorded and narrowly transcribed by a trained listener. From these samples, the learner's underlying representation of morphemes, and phonetic and phonemic inventories were determined, as well as the distribution of sounds, phonological rules, and phonotactic constraints.

Results of the analysis indicated that the learner had a relatively complete inventory of English sounds, and also used sounds common to Spanish but not English ([x], [β], and [ɣ]). The following rule-governed properties of the learner's IL were observed:

(1) an allophonic rule such that [b], [d], and [g] were in complementary distribution with [β], [ð], and [ɣ], respectively. The stops occurred word-initially and the fricatives, postvocalically;

(2) a positional constraint such that [z] did not occur in word-initial position; and

(3) an inventory constraint that excluded [v] in all word positions.

It was these three properties of the IL system that were examined experimentally as independent parameters to determine relative ease of phonological learning.

The learner exhibited an optional rule of terminal devoicing which was ordered before the rule of post-vocalic spirantization (1 above). The effects of this rule are not considered here since the errored sounds were trained in word-initial position only.

Experimental Design and Procedures

A single-subject multiple-baseline design across three behaviors was used (McReynolds and Kearns, 1983) whereby training began with one sound contrast and continued to predetermined levels of accuracy while the other two contrasts were monitored. Training then shifted to the next contrast with remaining contrasts monitored. This sequence of observation/training continued until all targeted contrasts were taught. Experimental control was demonstrated when changes only occurred during conditions of training, but not observation. As a further insurance of experimental control, two other sounds were monitored: /f/, a sound known and used target-appropriately, and [ɣ] a known but target-inappropriate sound. No changes in the learner's use of /f/ or [ɣ] served as an added demonstration of experimental control.

For this learner, three sound contrasts were selected for training from the errored aspects of the IL identified in the pretraining phonological analysis: /ð/ vs. /d/, /z/ vs. /s/, and /v/ vs. /b/. All contrasts were trained in word-initial position using minimal pairs, comprised of phonotactically permissible non-words depicted in pictures (see Appendix). For each targeted contrast, non-words represented four nouns, four verbs, and two adjectives, for a total of five minimal training pairs. Non-words have been used extensively and effectively in speech-language pathology (Gerber 1973; Gierut 1990; McDonald 1964; Powell and McReynolds 1969; VanRiper 1978; Winitz 1975) and psycholinguistic research (Foss and Swinney 1973; Morton and Long 1976; Rubin, Turvey, and VanGelder 1976), and more recently in studies of second language acquisition (Dickerson 1987). In the present study, non-words afforded carefully controlled contexts for training and insured that the learner was presented with the same task of learning "new" lexical items consisting of target-appropriate sounds previously used in error in his grammar.

Training of each contrast proceeded independently in the following order: overcoming the phonological rule, the positional constraint, and then the inventory constraint. Training began in an imitative mode and then continued in a spontaneous mode of production until the learner achieved 90% accurate production over two consecutive sessions in each mode. Productions were judged as accurate if the target sound was native-like; other sounds in the word did not have to be produced accurately. Once criterion was met in both modes, the pretraining picture naming protocol and a brief continuous speech sample were obtained to monitor changes in production and to establish relative ease of learning.

Reliability

To evaluate reliability of the phonetic transcriptions, 20% of the learner's single word utterances and 25% of his continuous speech were transcribed by a trained independent judge (SC). A point-to-point comparison of consonant transcriptions showed 87% agreement between the two judges for the learner's continuous speech, and 90% agreement for the single word utterances.

Results and Discussion

Relative ease of phonological learning was defined *a priori*: (1) learning during training, (2) generalization learning, and (3) learning that resulted in phonological restructuring. Each of these three aspects of learning will be examined in turn following from Figure 1. This figure shows percent target-appropriate productions of the trained contrasts in the trained word-initial position. Target sounds produced in error are marked with circles. Points to the left of the first dotted line show the multiple baseline sequence of each of the three trained contrasts prior to training, as measured in untrained real words. Only truly spontaneous productions were included in the baselines; responses elicited from delayed imitations were excluded. Points

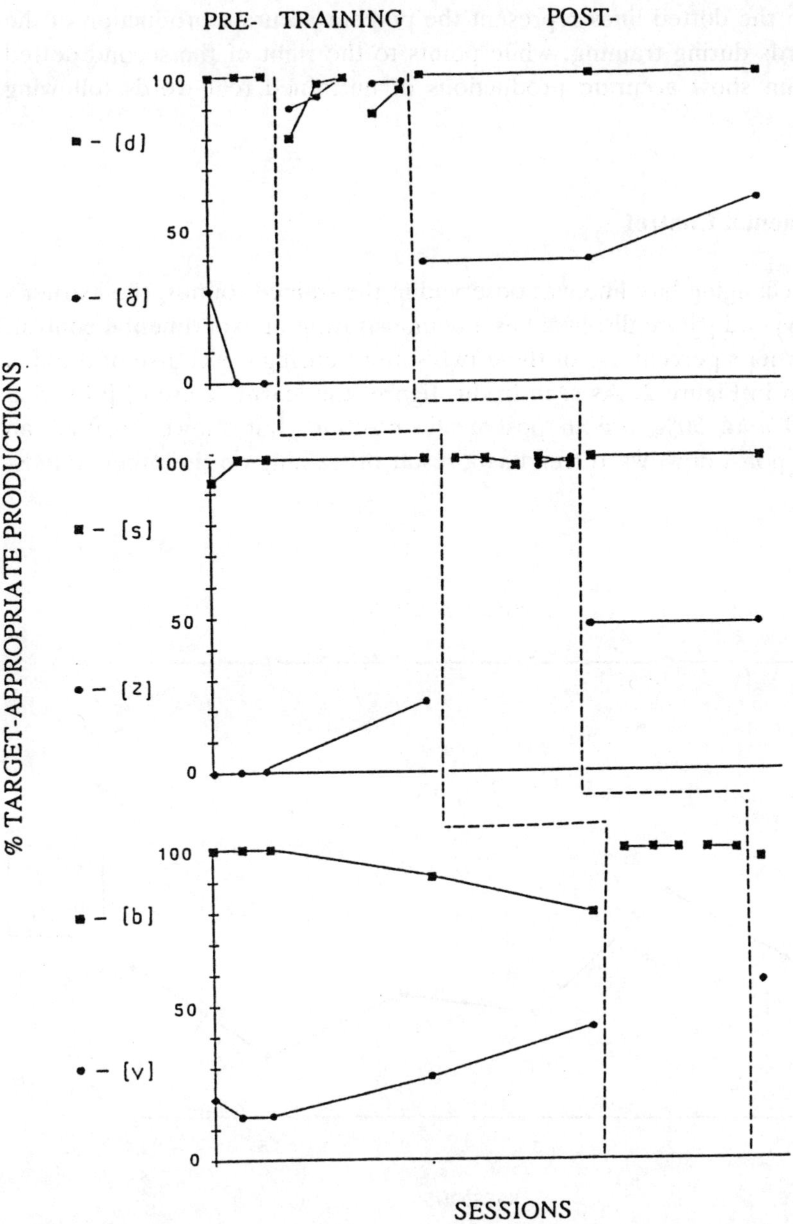

Figure 1. Percent target-appropriate productions of trained sounds in word-initial position over time.

between the dotted lines represent the percent accurate production of the non-words during training, while points to the right of the second dotted line again show accurate productions of untrained real words following training.

Experimental Control

Since a changing baseline was observed in the trained sounds, the learner's use of [γ] and [f] are displayed as a demonstration of experimental control. The learner's percent use of these two sounds during the course of training is shown in Figure 2. As seen in this figure, the learner's use of [γ] varied from 20% to 50% use in postvocalic position, but showed neither an upward nor a downward trend as a result of training on the other sounds.

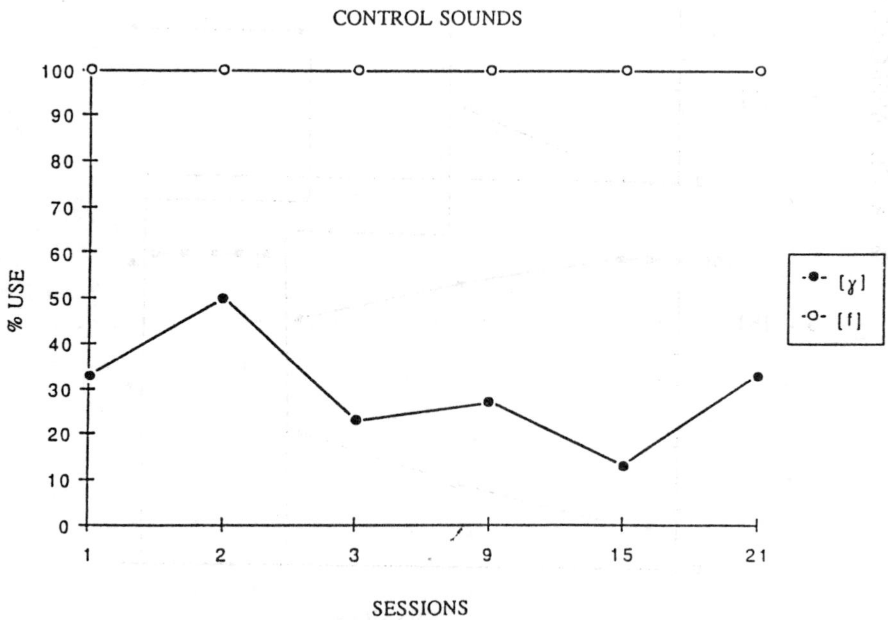

Figure 2. Percent use of control sounds. Points correspond in time to pre- and post-training sessions in Figure 1.

No changes were observed in the learner's use of [f], which was used with 100% accuracy throughout training. Hence, experimental control was demonstrated.

Learning During Training

The first measure for evaluating ease of phonological learning was learning during training. This measure consisted of an examination of the number of trials to criterion and percent accurate production of trained non-word minimal pairs. These factors were examined because, perhaps, contrasts that are easiest to learn would be mastered in fewer trials and to higher degrees of accuracy. It can be seen in Figure 1 that, with respect to trials to criterion, the learner achieved the predetermined criterion in the fewest possible training days for all three contrasts. Also, percent accurate production of trained items was at or near 100% accuracy for all three contrasts. Thus no differences in ease of learning emerged between the three phonological properties as measured by the subject's performance during training.

Although learning during training did not prove a relevant factor in determining ease of phonological learning for this subject, this finding is consistent with a recent study on phonologically disordered children by Gierut (1990). Gierut also observed no differences in performance across children during training and attributed these similarities to general cognitive constraints associated with memory of novel lexical items.

Generalization Learning

The second measure of ease of learning, generalization learning, focused on the learner's use of target sounds in the trained word-initial position in untrained real words. Generalization learning was evaluated since errored aspects of the phonology easiest to learn would presumably show the greatest change to untreated items without direct training. Comparing the learner's performance before and after training, all three trained sounds showed improvements. However, immediately following training, [ð] was used target-appropriately 40% of the time, [z] was used target-appropriately 50% of the time, and [v], 57% of the time. These data suggest, as a preliminary observation, that for this learner the inventory constraint excluding [v] was easier to overcome than the positional constraint involving [z], and that, in turn, was easier than the phonological rule affecting [ð]. It is of course possible that these findings were due to the cumulative effects of training since the allophonic rule involving [ð] was trained first and the inventory constraint involving /v/, last. To further validate these findings, a replication of this study across subjects is needed in which the order of training is reversed and counterbalanced. Nevertheless, this study provides preliminary evidence that an inventory constraint is easier to overcome than a positional constraint, which is, in turn, easier to overcome than an allophonic rule.

Phonological Restructuring

A final factor in determining ease of phonological learning was associated with restructuring of the learner's phonological system. Phonological restructuring was determined from a descriptive phonological analysis conducted immediately after training, employing the same procedures as in the pre-training analysis. It was predicted that the learner's overall phonological system would change to accommodate training such that errors would no longer be observed in sounds that were easier to learn. From the post-training analysis, several changes were observed with regard to the three trained phonological properties and each will be addressed in turn.

Prior to training, the learner exhibited an allophonic rule whereby [ð] and [d] were in complementary distribution. Following training, the learner used [ð] frequently and target-appropriately in word-initial position of spontaneous connected speech; post-vocalically, [ð] and [d] occurred in free variation. Although the changes in the learner's use of [ð] were not complete, they parallel those observed for phonologically disordered children learning to overcome allophonic rules (Gierut, 1986). For this group, following training, the phonological system was modified to include a phonemic contrast in one position along with position-specific free variation. As with phonologically disordered children, the L2 learner in this study would require further training on the [ð] - [d] contrast post-vocalically in order to induce a complete phonemic split.

The second errored aspect of this learner's system prior to training was a positional constraint which excluded [z] from word-initial position. Although [z] was used appropriately in the structured picture-naming protocol following training, the learner did not use [z] word-initially in continuous speech. It appears, then, that this sound was still excluded from word-initial position by a positional constraint in spite of direct training. However, since [z] does not occur frequently in word-initial position in English, it is possible that the learner simply did not have the opportunity to use the sound in his continuous speech.

Finally, the inventory constraint which excluded /v/ from all word positions prior to training was no longer evident in the post-training analysis. The learner used /v/ appropriately both word-initially and post-vocalically following training. Concomitant with this change, the allophonic relationship between [b] and [β] was no longer observed. The phoneme /b/ occurred post-vocalically following training, and [β] was no longer used. Interestingly, this change in the allophonic rule occurred *only* after training on the inventory constraint. The use of [b] and [β] did not change following direct training on the allophonic rule involving [d] and [ð]. This implies that training on the inventory constraint, in the contrast [v] vs. [b], had a double impact on the phonological system because it affected not only the inventory constraint but also the allophonic rule.

The data from phonological restructuring provide perhaps the strongest evidence that for this L2 learner the inventory constraint was easier to overcome than other errored aspects of his system. The inventory constraint was not only easier to overcome, but training on the inventory constraint was more effective since it resulted in broader changes in the learner's overall phonological system. The present study thus provides a second demonstration, following Hammerly (1982) and others (Flege, 1987; Valdman, 1976), that learning new sounds not previously in the inventory will be easier for L2 learners than overcoming other errored aspects of a phonological system. Importantly, this study allowed for heterogeneity across IL phonological systems in an experimental examination of ease of learning. This is in contrast to Hammerly's (1982) longitudinal descriptive study of ease of learning in which homogeneity among learners was assumed. Despite differences in methodologies and assumptions, the results of these two studies were consistent regarding ease of learning for L2. It is of interest that the present study differs from Gierut and Dinnsen (1987) for phonologically disordered children. These investigators found that inventory constraints were the most difficult to master. These conflicting findings raise the possibility that the course of language learning and ease of learning may differ for second language learners and speech disordered children.

Retention

A final result of this study relates to retention, an issue not widely examined in speech-language pathology or second language acquisition. To address this issue, the learner in this study was called back for an additional single word speech sample 3 1/2 weeks after training, following the same procedures described above. The results of this last speech sample are shown as a final data point added to the first figure, shown here as Figure 3. As seen in this figure, all three trained aspects of the learner's system returned to near 0% baseline levels after only 3 1/2 weeks without training. The learner was not producing any of the treated sounds — [ð], [z], or [v] — in the treated position. In spite of training and demonstrated improvements in performance immediately following training, the phonological changes observed were apparently only temporary.

This lack of retention raises important pedagogical and theoretical questions with regard to the restructuring of L2 sound systems. First, the lack of retention on the part of this L2 learner appears, on the surface, to negate the original findings of this study. How can it be claimed that certain aspects of the learner's phonology were easier to learn than others since improvements were not maintained in either case?

Here, it is necessary to emphasize the distinction between a demonstration of experimental effects versus a demonstration of ecological effects (cf. McReynolds and Kearns 1983). This study clearly demonstrated the experimental and controlled effects of phonological training. Without question, the learner's improvement in sound production was the result of training rather than extraneous influences. When training was withdrawn, improvements were no longer evidenced. The return to baseline established a direct cause-effect relationship between phonological change and training.

Yet, this learner's return to baseline levels raises serious questions about the ecological validity of intensive pronunciation training. Although the minimal pair training methods employed in this study resulted in immediate phonological improvements, these were only transient. Perhaps the minimal pair method of training actually constrained the more permanent integration of sounds in the phonology. Methods of L2 instruction need to be re-evaluated and new methods need to be developed to accommodate this problem. Perhaps less intensive, intermittent, or longer-term training would be more effective.

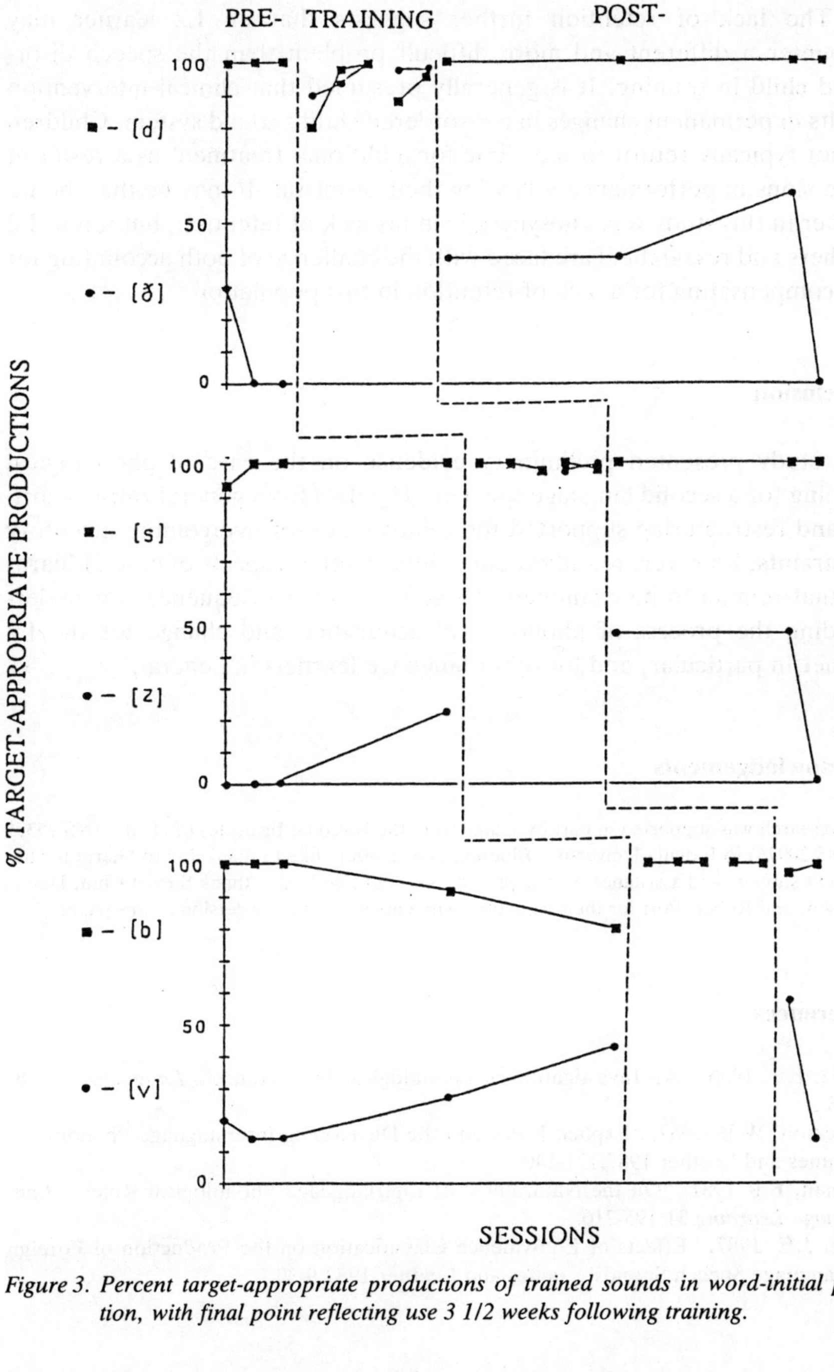

Figure 3. Percent target-appropriate productions of trained sounds in word-initial position, with final point reflecting use 3 1/2 weeks following training.

The lack of retention further suggests that an L2 learner may encounter a different and more difficult problem than the speech disordered child in training. It is generally presumed that clinical intervention results in permanent changes in a disordered child's sound system. Children do not typically return to the clinic for additional treatment as a result of regressions in performance following their dismissal. It may be that the L2 learner in this study was idiosyncratic in his lack of retention, but if not, L2 teachers and researchers are faced with the challenge of both accounting for and compensating for a lack of retention in this population.

Conclusion

This study presented preliminary evidence on the ease of phonological learning for a second language speaker. The data from generalization learning and restructuring supported the relative ease of overcoming inventory constraints; however, retention data identify other aspects of ease of learning that remain to be examined. These will have consequences for understanding the process of phonological acquisition and change for the L2 learner in particular, and for other language learners in general.

Acknowledgements

This research was supported in part by grants from the National Institutes of Health (NS 25375 and NS 20976) to Indiana University, Bloomington. I would like to thank Judith Gierut for her frequent support and assistance on this project. I would also like to thank Steven Chin, Daniel Dinnsen, and Robert Port for their valuable comments on an earlier version of this paper.

References

Brière, E.J. 1966. "An Investigation of Phonological Interference". *Language* 42.768-96.

Dickerson, W.B. 1987. "Explicit Rules and the Developing Interlanguage Phonology". James and Leather 1987.121-140.

Eckman, F.R 1981. "On the Naturalness of Interlanguage Phonological Rules". *Language Learning* 31.195-216.

Flege, J.E. 1987. "Effects of Equivalence Classification on the Production of Foreign Language Speech Sounds". James and Leather 1987.9-39.

Foss, D.J. and D.A. Swinney. 1973. "On the Psychological Reality of the Phoneme: Perception, Identification, and Consciousness". *Journal of Verbal Learning and Verbal Behavior* 12.246-257.

Gerber, A. 1973. *Goal: Carryover*. Philadelphia: Temple University Press.

Gierut, J.A. 1985. *On the relationship between phonological knowledge and generalization learning in misarticulating children*. Doctoral dissertation, Indiana University, Bloomington. Distributed by the Indiana University Linguistics Club, 1986.

Gierut, J.A. 1986. "Sound Change: A Phonemic Split in a Misarticulating Child". *Applied Psycholinguistics* 7.57-68.

Gierut, J.A. 1990. "Differntial Learning of Phonological Oppositions". *Journal of Speech and Hearing Research* 33.540-549.

Gierut, J.A. and D.A. Dinnsen. 1987. "On Predicting Ease of Phonological Learning". *Applied Linguistics* 8.241-63.

Hammerly, H. 1982. "Contrastive Phonology and Error Analysis". *International Review of Applied Linguistics* 20.17-32.

James, A. and J. Leather, eds. 1987. *Sound Patterns in Second Language Acquisition*. Dordrecht: Foris.

Kenstowicz, M. and C. Kisseberth. 1979. *Generative Phonology: Description and Theory*. New York: Academic Press, Inc.

McDonald, F.I. 1964. *Screening Deep Test of Articulation*. Pittsburgh: Stanwix House.

McReynolds, L.V. and K.P. Kearns. 1983. *Single-subject Experimental Designs in Communicative Disorders*. Baltimore: University Park Press.

Morton, J. and J. Long. 1976. "Effect of Word Transitional Probability on Phoneme Identification". *Journal of Verbal Learning and Verbal Behavior* 12.431-461.

Powell, J. and L.V. McReynolds. 1969. "A Procedure for Testing Position Generalization from Articulation Training". *Journal of Speech and Hearing Research* 12.629-644.

Rubin, P., M.T. Turvey and P. VanGelder. 1976. "Initial Phonemes Are Detected Faster in Spoken Words Than in Spoken Nonwords". *Perception & Psychophysics* 19.394-398.

Valdman, A. 1976. *Introduction to French Phonology and Morphology*. Rowley, MA: Newbury House.

VanRiper, C. 1978. *Speech Correction: Principles and Methods*. Englewood Cliffs, NJ: Prentice-Hall.

Winitz, H. 1975. *From Syllable to Conversation*. Baltimore: University Park Press.

Appendix

Non-word minimal pairs used in training.

[d] vs. [ð]	[s] vs. [z]	[b] vs. [v]
1. [dipəl] ~ [ðipəl]	1. [sikəl ~ [zikəl]	1. [bɛŋ] ~ [vɛŋ]
2. [dɛč] ~ [ðɛč]	2. [sičəm] ~ [zičəm]	2. [bɔklɩŋ] ~ [vɔkliŋ]
3. [dump] ~ [ðump]	3. [sɛkər] ~ [zɛkər]	3. [bɔnči] ~ [vɔnči]
4. [dik] ~ [ðik]	4. [suk] ~ [zuk]	4. [bɛnəl] ~ [vɛnəl]
5. [dupi] ~ [ðupi]	5. [sɛpi] ~ [zɛpi]	5. [buč] ~ [vuč]

Acquisition and Loss of Familiar Language:

Idiom and Proverb Comprehension

Daniel Kempler and Diana Van Lancker
University of Southern California

Introduction

Some language is familiar. Familiar language, including proverbs ("Rome wasn't built in a day"), idioms ("He kicked the bucket") and social interaction formulas ("Catch you later") have been largely ignored by linguists. Rather, linguists have focused their attention on the structure and meaning of novel utterances (e.g. "The president ran the hundred mile race carrying the baboon on his back"). However, the familiar (memorized) aspects of language contribute importantly to native-like fluency, allowing utterances and conversations to flow smoothly.

Linguists (e.g. Weinreich 1969), psychologists (Gorham 1956; Swinney and Cutler 1979) and speech pathologists (Nippold, Martin and Erstine 1988) have approached the issue of familiar language from different vantage points, all reaching various conclusions. For example, some linguists and experimental psychologists have argued that familiar phrases are structurally and semantically like single words. On the other hand, developmental psychologists have demonstrated that familiar phrases are learned much later than other aspects of language, and not mastered until the late teen years, which contrasts directly with the single-word hypothesis. In addition, clinicians, particularly neurologists and psychiatrists, routinely use familiar language to aid in the diagnosis of psychiatric and neurological disorders, although there is little evidence that we understand the neurology of familiar language nearly as well as we understand the lateralization and localization of other aspects of language within the brain.

Part of the difficulty in developing a coherent picture of the nature of familiar language has been a lack of a simple protocol which can be used with various populations — especially with children and those with brain injury. Some of these prior investigations have been beset by methodological problems. For instance, a common method of assessing proverb comprehension is to ask people to verbally interpret a selected proverb. This is of questionable validity with a number of populations: children have difficulty giving definitions of even single words long after they "understand" them; brain-injured people may not be able to verbalize much at all, but may have intact comprehension. In studying familiar language, other studies have confused newly created metaphoric language with familiar language, which is known to be learned by children at different rates (Pollio and Pollio 1974) and are probably processed differently by adults. Other methodological problems include the lack of control sentences (i.e. children and patients are never asked to "interpret" non-familiar sentences) and the failure to establish whether subjects are familiar with the test items.

In order to circumvent some of these methodological problems, we have developed a simple picture-pointing comprehension task using familiar proverbs, idioms and speech formulas suitable for many populations. The goal of the research has been to develop such a protocol and to systematically assess comprehension of familiar and novel language by normal and language-disordered children, non-native English speakers and individuals with focal and diffuse brain injury as part of developing a coherent theory of how familiar language is learned, used and processed by the brain.

Methods

The *Familiar and Novel Language Comprehension* (FANL-C) protocol was developed to require no verbal output and little or no metalinguistic functioning — only a pointing response is needed. The patient is shown a set of four line drawings and asked to select the one that matches a sentence read aloud by the examiner. There are 40 test items: 20 familiar phrases, including proverbs ("While the cat's away, the mice will play"), idioms ("That's enough to drive a man to drink"), and contextually bound social interaction formulas ("I'll get back to you later"). All familiar items were selected to be common, picturable, familiar and easily recognized by normal adults. The novel sentences were constructed to match the familiars in overall length (number of words), surface grammatical structure, and word-frequency. The foils (wrong answers) included no "literal" meanings (since

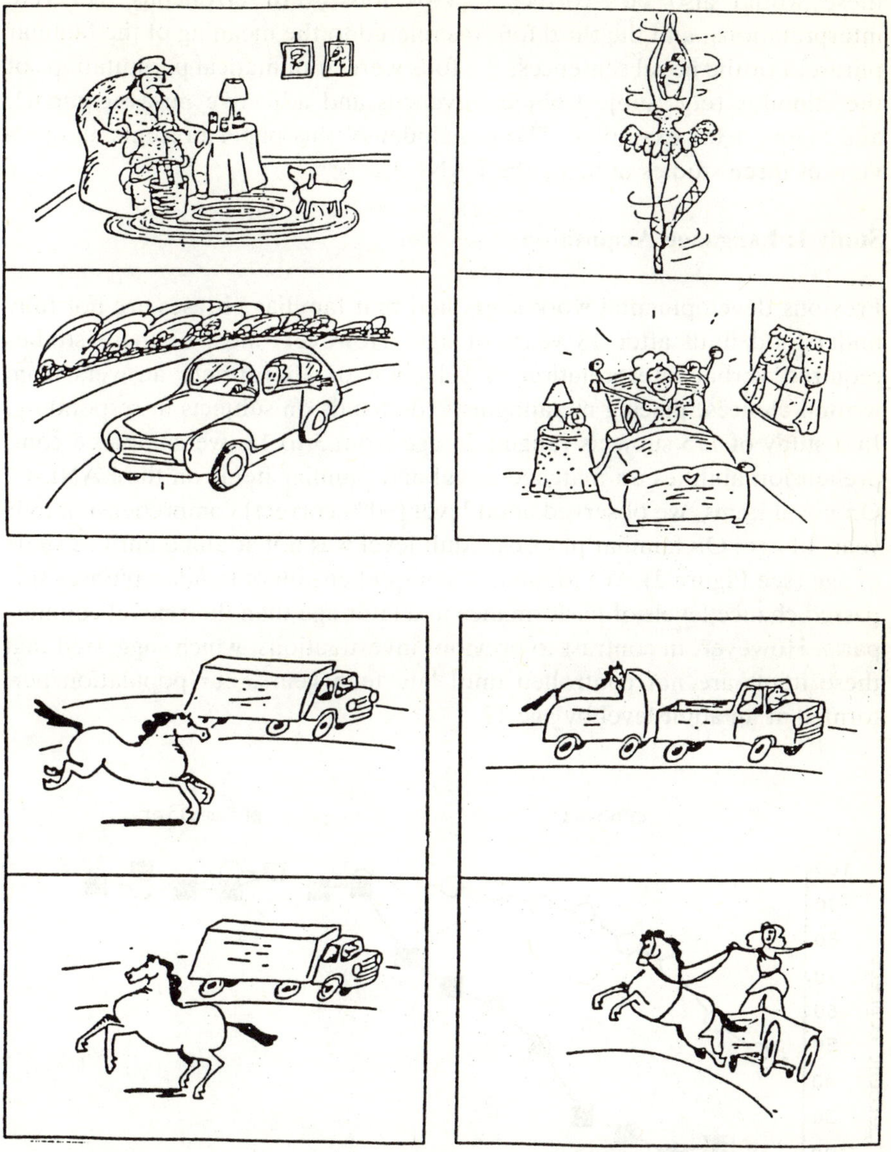

Figure 1. Sample picture arrays for familiar (top) and novel (bottom) stimuli. Top: "She took a sudden turn for the worse." Bottom: "He's racing a truck against a horse."

these would also be "correct"). Two foils were erroneous, concrete interpretations, and the third foil was related to the meaning of the familiar phrase. For the novel sentences, the foils were grammatical permutations of the stimulus (e.g. subject-object reversals and adjective misassignment). See Figure 1 for examples. The remainder of this paper presents an overview of three studies utilizing the FANL-C.

Study 1: Language Acquisition

Previous developmental work suggested that familiar phrases are not fully understood until after 18 years of age. However, most of these studies required verbal interpretation or selection of appropriate answers from written choices, placing metalinguistic demands on subjects in responding. In a study of 175 subjects ranging in age from 3 to 18, we compared comprehension abilities on matched novel and familiar items on the FANL-C. On novel items, we observed adult level (90% correct) comprehension by 8 years of age. On familiar phrases, adult level was not attained until 12 years of age (see Figure 2). We found that comprehension of familiar phrases surpassed chance levels of performance at a later age than their novel counterparts. However, in contrast to previous investigations, which suggested that these items are not controlled until late teen years, our population performed at an adult level by age 12.

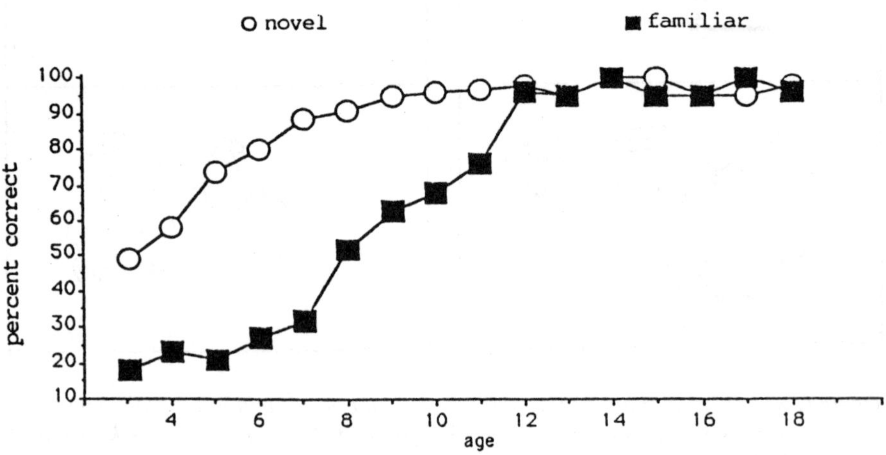

Figure 2. Comprehension (percent correct) of familiar and novel phrases for subjects age 3-18.

Study 2: Left vs. Right Brain Damage

It has long been suggested that familiar language may be represented in both cerebral hemispheres, while novel language is generally restricted to the dominant (left) hemisphere. The data supporting differential representation of novel vs. familiar language has come mostly from observations that language appears to be relatively spared in cases of aphasia due to left

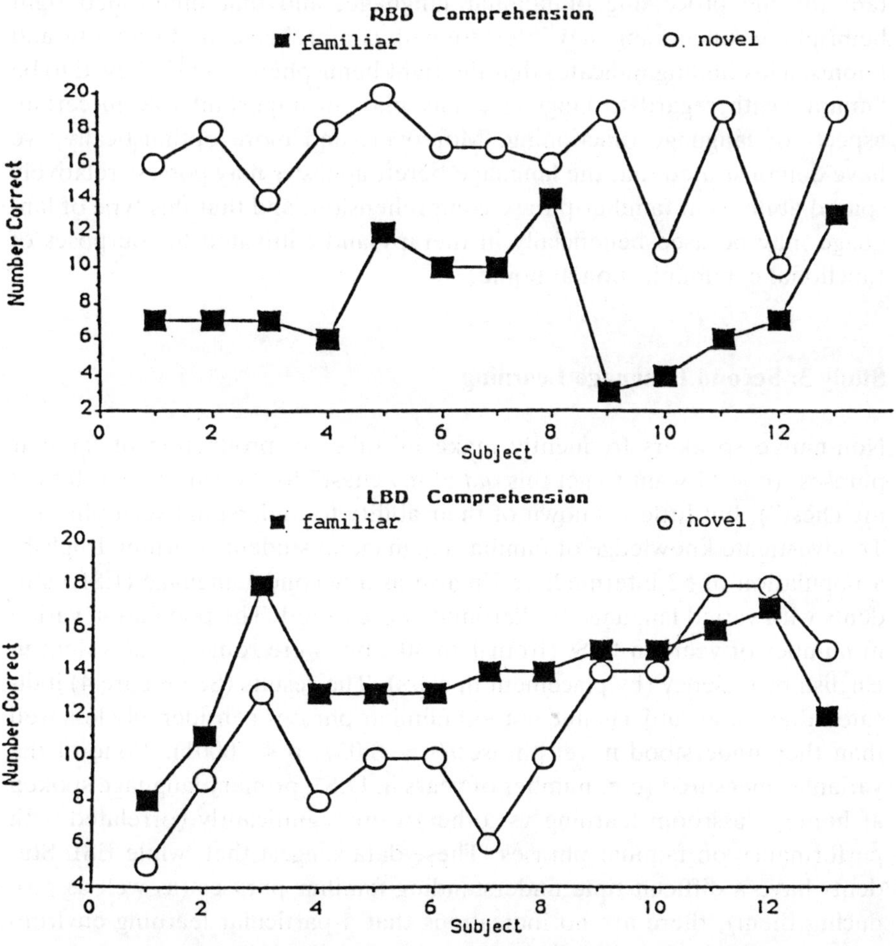

Figure 3. Percent correct comprehension of familiar and novel phrases for right- (top) and left-(bottom) brain damaged patients.

hemisphere lesions. A published study (VanLancker and Kempler 1987) using an earlier version of the FANL-C indicated that right brain damaged patients uniformly performed worse on familiar than novel phrases. Using the revised FANL-C, these findings were replicated on 13 unilateral left- and 13 unilateral right-brained injured patients. Eleven of the 13 left brain damaged aphasics performed better on familiar than novel phrases. In both studies statistical analyses revealed a significant effect of task, group and a group x task interaction ($p < .001$).

These data suggest that the non-dominant right hemisphere is important for the processing of familiar language, and that diminished right hemisphere functioning may interfere with comprehension of proverbs and idioms. This finding indicates that the right hemisphere, long believed to be "minor" with regard to language, may play an important role in certain aspects of language functioning. Moreover, and more optimistically, we have demonstrated that the language-bereft aphasics may possess relatively spared abilities in familiar phrase comprehension, and that this type of language may be used beneficially in therapy and cultivated for purposes of functional communication at home.

Study 3: Second Language Learning

Non-native speakers frequently make mistakes in production of familiar phrases, (e.g. "I want to get this *out* of my chest" for "I want to get this *off* my chest"), but little is known of their ability to understand such phrases. To investigate knowledge of familiar language in students learning English, a population of 52 intermediate English as a Second Language (ESL) students with varied language backgrounds were tested. The population varied in number of years in U.S. (from 1 to 40), but were roughly equivalent in English proficiency (by placement in class). The results (See Figure 4) indicated that these subjects understood familiar phrases considerably less well than they understood novel phrases ($t = 8.037$, $p < .0001$). None of the variables measured (e.g. number of years in U.S., primary language spoken at home, classroom learning vs. other) were significantly correlated with performance on familiar phrases. These data suggest that, while ESL Students have a difficult time understanding familiar phrases (as well as producing them), there are no indications that a particular learning environment contributes to the ability to learn these difficult items.

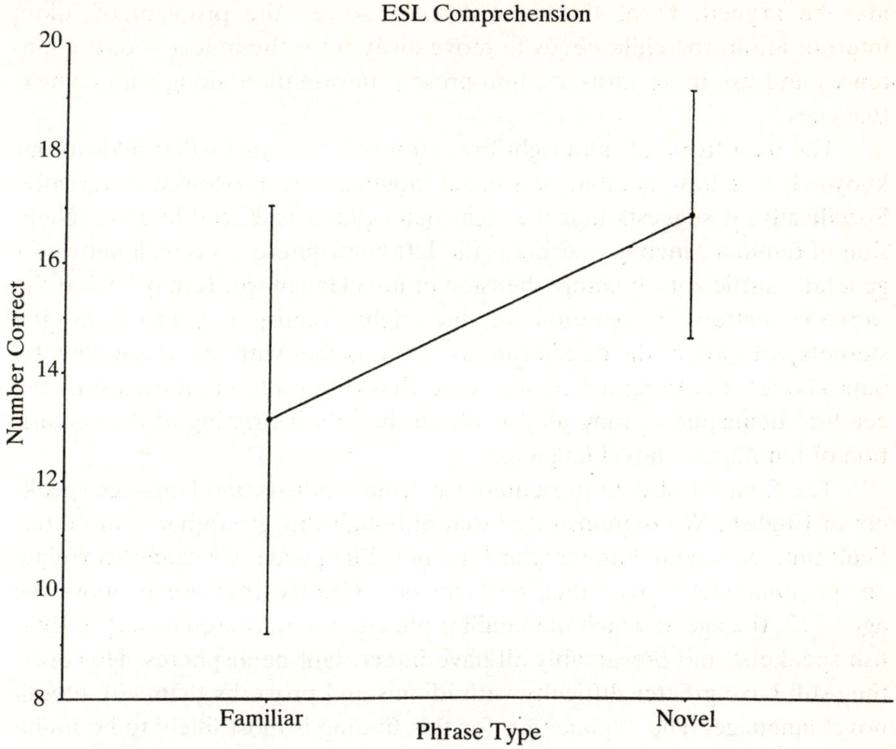

Figure 4. Mean number correct (with standard deviation bars) for familiar and novel phrases by 52 ESL students.

Discussion

By investigating three distinct populations with a single, carefully designed comprehension test, we have begun to fill in the gaps in our knowledge about familiar language. In language development, it appears that familiar language is acquired at a slower pace than novel language, not appearing until about age 8, and reaching an adult level by 12 years. Cognitive developments that take place between 7 and 9 (e.g. concrete operational thought may be important for mastering these aspects of language. The development of concrete operational thought allows children to move away from simple perceptual observations of problems, and solve problems with information that is not an easily observed perceptual feature of an object. It may be argued, then, that in order to "solve" the problem of idiom interpretation, the child needs to move away from the object (i.e. the sentence) and use more abstract, non-present information along with contextual cues.

The data from left and right brain injured patients further adds to our knowledge of how familiar and novel language are processed differently. Specifically, it suggests that the right hemisphere is crucial in comprehension of familiar language, whereas the left hemisphere, as is well known, is generally sufficient for comprehension of novel language. It may be that the superior pattern recognition of the right hemisphere processes the stereotyped form of the familiar items. Put together with the developmental data above, it is tempting to speculate that differential maturation of the cerebral hemispheres may play a role in the relative timing of the acquisition of familiar vs. novel language.

The final bit of data presented was from adult second language speakers of English. We demonstrated that although this group had a more difficult time understanding familiar than novel language, we cannot correlate any personal factors with their performance. Clearly, they are all above the age of 12, the age at which the familiar phrases are mastered by native English speakers, and presumably all have intact right hemispheres. However, they still have greater difficulty with idioms and proverbs than with literal/novel language. The explanation for this finding is most likely to be found in the properties of familiar language. There are thousands of familiar phrases and each is made up of a stereotyped form and a conventional meaning whose appropriate use is tightly tied to a range of particular contexts. This information is difficult to teach formally, and learning them as an adult most likely depends on exposure to the phrases in sufficiently clear contexts to extract the crucial meaning.

The cognitive and neurological mechanism by which familiar phrases are learned and processed remain poorly understood. Yet familair language is an important component of linguistic ability worthy of careful, thorough study. We offer the FANL-C and these preliminary investigations as first steps in the study of familiar language comprehension.

References

Gorham, D.R. 1956. "A Proverbs Test for Clinical and Experimental Use". *Psychological Reports* 1.1-12.

Nippold, M.A, S.A. Martin and B.J. Erskine. 1988. "Proverb Comprehension in Context: A Developmental Study with Children and Adolescents". *Journal of Speech and Hearing Research* 3.19-28.
Pollio, M.R. and H.R. Pollio. 1974. "The Development of Figurative Language in Children". *Journal of Psycholinguistic Research* 3.195-201.
Swinney, D.A. and A. Cutler. 1979. "The Access and Processing of Idiomatic Expression". *Journal of Verbal Learning and Verbal Behavior* 18.523-534.
Van Lancker, D. and D. Kempler. 1987. "Comprehension of Familiar Phrases by Left- But Not by Right-Hemisphere Damaged Patients". *Brain and Language* 32.265-277.

Subject Index

In the series LANGUAGE ACQUISITION AND LANGUAGE DISORDERS (LALD) the following titles have been published:

1. WHITE, Lydia: *Universal Grammar Second Language Acquisition*. Amsterdam/Philadelphia, 1989.
2. HUEBNER, Thom and Charles A. FERGUSON (eds): *Crosscurrents in Second Language Acquisition and Linguistic Theories*. Amsterdam/Philadelphia, 1991.
3. EUBANK, Lynn (ed.): *Point-Counter-Point. Universal Grammar and Second Language Acquisition*. Amsterdam/Philadelphia, 1991.
4. ECKMAN, Fred R. (ed.): *Confluence. Linguistics, L2 acquisition and speech pathology*. Amsterdam/Philadelphia, 1993.
5. GASS, Susan and Larry SELINKER (eds): *Language Transfer in Language Learning*. Amsterdam/Philadelphia, 1992.